HEALTHY BODY; HEALTHY HAIR

A Natural Guide to Healthy Hair
and Hair Loss Prevention

Ken Peters - Nick Waddell

Apple Tree Publishing Company Ltd.
VANCOUVER CANADA

WWW.APPLEPUBLISHING.COM

Copyright 2007 by Ken Peters and Nick Waddell

Apple Tree Publishing Company Ltd. reserves all rights to this edition. No part of this work may be reproduced or transmitted in any form or by any means, electronic or mechanical, including photocopying and recording, or by any information storage or retrieval system, except for those wishing to quote brief passages in connection with a review.

The information contained in this book was prepared from sources which are believed to be accurate and reliable. However, the opinions expressed herein by the author(s) do not necessarily represent the opinions or the views of the publisher. Readers are strongly advised to seek the advice of their personal health care professional(s) before proceeding with any changes in any health care program.

Library and Archives Canada Cataloguing in Publication

Peters, Ken, 1956-
    Healthy body, healthy hair : a natural guide to healthy hair and hair loss prevention / Ken Peters, Nick Waddell.

Includes bibliographical references.

ISBN 978-1-896817-30-9

    1. Baldness--Prevention. 2. Hair--Care and hygiene. 3. Health. I. Waddell, Nick II. Title.

RL91.P47 2007   616.5'46   C2007-900593-4

Apple Tree Publishing Company Ltd.
Vancouver, British Columbia CANADA

Printed in Hong Kong

TABLE OF CONTENTS

INTRODUCTION

CHAPTER ONE
Your Hair..1

CHAPTER TWO
Causes of Hair Loss..5

CHAPTER THREE
The Prostate and Male Pattern Baldness...............9

CHAPTER FOUR
Dietary Cocerns...13

CHAPTER FIVE
Vitamins...19

CHAPTER SIX
Minerals...29

CHAPTER SEVEN
Essential Fatty Acids...37

CHAPTER EIGHT
Juices...41

CHAPTER NINE
Circulation...45

CHAPTER TEN
Herbs & Plants: External Use...............................49

CHAPTER ELEVEN
Devices and Gadgets..59

CHAPTER TWELVE
Choosing a Shampoo & Conditioner.................................61

CHAPTER THIRTEEN
Washing Drying and Brushing..65

CHAPTER FOURTEEN
Nasty Chemicles...69

CHAPTER FIFTEEN
The Oriental Approach..75

CONCLUSION..83

BIBLIOGRAPHY..87

Introduction

AMERICAN MEDICAL ASSOCIATION figures show that forty per cent of all men will experience some degree of hair loss by the time they're forty. The number rises to sixty five per cent by the time they reach seventy. The figures are alarmingly high for women, as well.

These numbers sound familiar, even acceptable to our ears. Yet simple cross-cultural and historical comparison reveals that few societies rival ours when it comes to the attention given to hair loss.

It is at first glance, a seemingly trivial cosmetic change. Some men even feel they look better without hair. For most however, it is important. Important enough to sustain the four billion dollar industry that hair loss is here in North America.

If in terms of physical health, hair loss were an isolated phenomenon concerning only the health of follicles and scalp, it would likely still be a four billion dollar industry. The condition is infrequently linked to general health in our society. Perhaps we have made an unconscious assumption that nothing can be done. If so, this is unfortunate. For perspective and examination consistently point to poor hair health and hair loss as symptomatic of larger, broader based lifestyle-related problems. Diet is the most dramatic and influential of these, and as such, is our primary focus.

For comparison's sake we will detail a few conventional treatments for hair loss.

Introduction

One of the more popular procedures is the hair transplant. During a hair transplant small pieces of skin containing tufts of hair are removed from the back and sides of the head. These 'plugs' are then surgically inserted into the thinning areas at a cost of thousands of dollars, depending on how many plugs must be inserted. Unfortunately, the quality of the finished product can vary greatly; much depends upon the skill of the surgeon. In order for the job to appear natural the surgeon must possess both good surgical technique and artistic ability.

Another specialized surgical procedure known as scalp reduction has been used with some success. In a series of operations the scalp is cut and a section of flesh is shifted forward to cover balding areas. The patient must wear a dressing until the scalp heals and then, usually about six weeks later, the operation is repeated. The process often takes more than a year to complete.

A new technique currently popular is the hair weave, which is the least invasive (i.e. non-surgical) of the cosmetic cover-ups. Here real hair of the same color is woven into one's hair base until the balding area is hidden. It will last for months through regular activities and then must be upgraded. Some patients find the weave to be irritating and unnatural.

The only product sanctioned by the USFDA and Health and Welfare Canada as a hair loss treatment is Minoxidil. Originally created as a high blood pressure medication by Upjohn Pharmaceuticals, researchers observed that it caused patients to sprout hair all over their bodies. Originally produced in tablet form the medicine was reformulated into a lotion called Rogaine, which received FDA approval in 1988. In July 1989, the FDA banned all non-prescription creams and lotions that claimed to cure or prevent baldness.

Because Rogaine, even applied topically, still has the potential to alter a user's blood pressure it is available only with a doctor's prescription. Rogaine is designed to be applied to the scalp twice a day at a cost of at least sixty dollars per month. In order for the product to be effective one

Introduction

must continue to use the product forever, or the resulting new growth will eventually fall out.

Dr. Shapiro, a dermatologist specializing in hair loss research and treatment at the University of British Columbia's Adult Hair Clinic claims that about thirty per cent of users will grow new hair, but only eight per cent of that hair is 'cosmetically acceptable.'

Even if one ignores the cost and associative difficulties of using Rogaine the risk of side effects is considerable. Upjohn itself has warned of possible negative side effects including 'increased heart rate, rapid weight gain or edema, difficulty in breathing, worsening of or new onset of angina pectoris.'

Many other potential side effects are mentioned, which along with those mentioned above, have been reported in the users of the tablet form prescribed to lower blood pressure. Even though the dosage is much lower in the topical solution it will still enter the bloodstream via the skin of the scalp.

The remedies in this book gathered from around the world -from the pages of tradition, history and science, share the distinction of being free of negative side effects. In fact, many of them offer positive health benefits. Some of these products, such as Polysorbate 80 and Biotin have shown to be effective at halting, even reversing hair loss in scientific double blind studies. Still, manufacturers of these products may make no legal claims as to their effectiveness.

This situation exists because the law requires that in order to claim that a product will 'cure' an ailment one must first obtain FDA approval (in Canada Health and Welfare). Obtaining such approval is a lengthy, expensive and somewhat political proposition, requiring extensive scientific experimentation and study -and the cost of such procedures are often in the hundreds of thousands of dollars.

Introduction

This kind of investment is only warranted when a company can obtain an exclusive patent on a given product that can guarantee a return on investment and a profit level worthy of the financial risk involved.

No one can control the rights to common substances such as vitamins (biotin), food emulsifiers (polysorbate 80), and herbs. Only drugs fall into this category.

The bottom line is this: if you are already bald there is probably very little you can do to reverse it naturally. However, this book will best benefit those with thinning hair, or those interested in prevention.

And as an added bonus, all who use the techniques and methods prescribed in this book will follow a safe path towards improving their general health and overall quality of life.

Not too bad a side effect! *-The Authors*

CHAPTER 1 Your Hair

THE SCALP IS A COMPLEX ORGAN containing between 100,000 and 150,000 hair follicles, an equal number of pigment and sebaceous glands, and thousands of sweat glands. There are at least half a million glands in the scalp that serve the purpose of growing hair, and to function properly they must be well nourished. *Starve these glands and hair loss begins.*

The development of hair starts when epidermal cells form a follicle: a hollow, cylindrical depression in the skin or scalp. Follicles produce Keratin, a protein comprised of carbon, hydrogen, nitrogen, sulfur and oxygen, which forms ninety seven per cent of the hair- shaft. The rest of the shaft is moisture. Hair, especially if brittle or thin, is sensitive enough to act as a natural barometer. In humid conditions it can absorb up to forty per cent of its' own weight in water.

Hair development goes through three stages: **anagen**, the growing stage, **catagen**, the transitional state, and **telogen**, the resting state. At any given time approximately eighty-five per cent of the hair is in the growing stage, fifteen per cent is the resting state. Each individual hair may grow for two to six years, then the follicle goes into a resting phase for about three months, during which there is no growth. When the hair follicle begins production again it starts to grow a new hair shaft, which pushes the old one out. Normally one loses fifty to a hundred hairs per day, and ideally gains the same number of new ones.

Sebaceous glands within follicles lubricate the scalp and hair with an oily, rich, yellowish substance called sebum. With its' ability to absorb and

CHAPTER 1 / Your Hair

retain large amounts of moisture, the sebum also fills skin tissue, keeping it plump and firm. A deficiency of sebum leads to a scalp that becomes dry and scaly; without it hair becomes brittle, and may break or split. An excess of sebum has also been linked to hair loss (see chapter 7: 'Essential Fatty Acids'). The sebaceous glands require Essential Fatty Acids in combination with a variety of minerals to produce sebum.

Once hair is visible it is literally dead tissue (much like fingernails). Hence, it is unable to repair itself, leaving it vulnerable to permanent damage. The only growing or live portion of the hair is its' root, which is located at the base of the follicle.

Cross Section of the Scalp fig 1

- External Hair
- Epidermis
- Hair Shaft
- Sabaceous Gland
- Matrix
- Bulb
- Dermal Papilla
- Fat Layer
- Epicranial Aponeurosis
- Connective Tissue
- Skull

The root envelops a tiny bulb-shaped organ called the papilla (the hair bud) which is filled with capillaries that deliver nutrients to the hair. The papilla are present at birth and each grows a couple of hairs. When you lose one, that hair is gone forever, much like a tooth. Both Iron and Iodine help the glands provide nourishment to the papilla.

The hair shaft consists of three layers: the medulla (inner layer), the cortex (middle layer), and the cuticle (outer covering). The medulla is the core of the shaft. As well as absorbing beneficial substances it serves as the supporting structure for the strand of hair. The cortex, protected by the cuticle, consists of rope-like protein fibers and hair color pigments. If the cuticle is damaged, the cortex is exposed allowing for moisture loss. The cortex then unravels in split ends and mid-shaft damage, which can lead to breakage. The cuticle is made of hard, transparent cells that overlap each other like the scales of a fish. These cells called imbrications are hinged, to open and close.

When these overlapping cells lie flat the hair feels smooth and looks shiny. Since it is the cuticle that gives elasticity and resiliency to the hair, its condition largely determines the hair's appearance. Hair growth in humans averages about one one-hundredth of an inch per day, and according to the scientific community does not grow faster when it is cut.

However, hair length may influence the rate of growth, slowing down once the length exceeds ten inches. Hair grows fastest in the summer and slowest in the winter. Growth speeds up under heat and friction (massage), but slows down when exposed to long periods of cold. The structure and strength of a gray hair is no different from that of a colored hair, and while the beginning of graying often corresponds with the start of hair loss, there is no evidence linking the two.

CHAPTER 2 Causes of Hair Loss

THINNING HAIR, a withering of the hair in its' follicle, can begin at any age after puberty. It can precede actual baldness by ten years or more (in which the follicle atrophies and stops producing hair altogether). Alopecia (the medical term for baldness or hair loss) is believed to be hereditary and generally incurable. The idea that nutritional deficiencies and inherited eating patterns actually create this condition has received very little research or support in the west. The fact that, for example, blond haired men are more predisposed to baldness than dark haired men, or Caucasians more than Blacks or Asians, is often attributed to genetic factors. However, investigation on the subject suggests that diet, nutrition and the environment may play a far greater role than previously suspected.

What is commonly referred to as Male Pattern Baldness was recognized as far back as the time of Hippocrates. He observed that castrated males would never go bald. Further on, it was discovered that balding men who were castrated as a result of wounds received during World War Two often regained their hair. More recently, studies have shown that such males, who no longer produce significant levels of testosterone, will sometimes lose their hair after being injected with androgens (male hormones). Interestingly, as soon as the injections were stopped, the patients regained their hair.

To understand how Male Pattern Baldness works it is first important to become familiar with the hormones involved. There are two types of sex hormones: estrogen, produced primarily in the ovaries, and androgens, the

CHAPTER 2 / Causes of Hair Loss

male specific hormones produced mostly in the testicles, predominantly in the form of testosterone. Testosterone is of special importance. Certain hair follicle cells are genetically predetermined to accept testosterone, while others are not. A limited amount of both types of hormone is also produced by the adrenal glands. It is this additional hormonal activity of the adrenals that can trigger hair loss.

Male Pattern Baldness is seen as operating on a biological clock. It is understood that hair follicles have a growing and resting cycle. When testosterone enters the follicles of those genetically predisposed to MPB, the hair follicles noticeable increase their production of the enzyme Testosterone 5-alpha Reductase.

In turn, this enzyme converts testosterone to a hormone called Dihydrotestosterone (DHT). Follicles exposed to DHT enter the resting phase and begin to atrophy and shrink. At the same time the galea aponeurotica membrane in the scalp becomes thickened and inelastic, cutting off circulation. In time the follicle structure becomes so withered and shallow, the scalp can no longer sustain hair growth. The hair growth cycle is altered and follicles begin to spend more time in the resting phase and less in the growing phase. Hair continues to fall out at the normal rate, but it is not replaced. Eventually there are no macroscopic hairs left in the area (the atrophied follicles are not necessarily dead however, and may be induced to resume growth with proper stimulation).

The adrenal hormones protect the body in stressful situations through the 'fight or flight' response. Adrenaline is released into the bloodstream, increasing heart rate, blood pressure and energy levels. In this heightened state the body is better able to deal with threatening situations. However, the body is unable to distinguish between these acute threats and the long-term stresses associated with modern life. Over time, this raises blood pressure and blood fat levels, increasing the risk of heart attack or stroke. Muscles and bones are weakened and the immune system is impaired.

Over-stimulated adrenal glands also produce extra androgens, thereby raising testosterone levels. Steroid hormones such as testosterone are made

CHAPTER 2 / Causes of Hair Loss

from cholesterol, a substance naturally present in the body. When steroid hormones are needed, additional cholesterol is drawn from the circulation, converted to the hormone, and quickly reintroduced to the bloodstream. A high intake of animal foods, notably dairy products, eggs and fatty meats, brings an excess of cholesterol into the body. The mechanism of constantly stressed adrenal glands combined with excess cholesterol can lead to the high level of androgens that is associated with Male Pattern Baldness.

After menopause many women will experience symptoms of hair loss, as well as an increased amount of facial hair. When a woman enters into menopause, or loses her period due to high level of physical activity or diet-

Cross Section of the Hair Follicle fig 2

The three stage of development of the Hair Follicle are:
Anagen (growth)   B) Catagen (transition) C) Telogen (rest).

The follicle stops producing a hair at the Telogen stage.
At this point, it shrivels up, and the bulb largely degenerates.

CHAPTER 2 / Causes of Hair Loss

ing, her estrogen levels drop.

Estrogen binds excess testosterone to proteins called globulins and lowers the free-form testosterone levels in the blood. Lowered levels of estrogen thus allow free testosterone levels to rise, leading to hair loss by the same mechanism as Male Pattern Baldness. The fine vellus hairs of the body, which are colorless and soft, are also converted into terminal hairs, which are coarser and pigmented.

A withdrawal from birth control pills, as well as childbirth, will cause a fall in estrogen levels. Hair loss after childbirth will return to normal levels after a few months. When the ovaries reduce their production of estrogen, as well as the related female hormone progesterone, the body is usually able to compensate by producing the required hormones through the adrenal glands.

However, when the body is overstressed and the adrenal glands are exhausted this backup system is insufficient. In this way the connection between the adrenal system and hair loss is as significant for women as it is for men. It is interesting to note that the conventional problems associated with menopause in the western world are uncommon in Japan. Because until recently, red meat (which raises testosterone levels) was rarely consumed by the Japanese, and soy foods (which contain estrogen like substances) were widely consumed.

The women of Japan were able to maintain high enough estrogen levels after menopause to avert menopausal problems.

CHAPTER 3 The Prostate and Male Pattern Baldness

THE PROSTATE is a cluster of small, doughnut-shaped sex glands. They encircle the urethra (the tube which conveys urine and semen) just below the bladder. Though all the functions of the prostate are not yet clear, its' most direct purpose is to contract during ejaculation. It squeezes the seminal fluid into and through the urethra tract. Because the prostate is located so close to the urethra, any problem with the prostate can hinder the free flow of urine.

It is interesting to note that as little as hundred years ago prostate problems were rarely mentioned in medical literature. This implies a link to a modern lifestyle (i.e. diet). Indeed, the connection between prostate cancer and a diet high in animal fats has been clearly established. About fifty per cent of men between the ages of forty and sixty have the most common disorder of the prostate gland: benign prostatic hyperplasia (BPH). Symptoms of BPH include increased frequency of urination, waking at night to empty the bladder, and reduced force and caliber of urination.

BPH is believed to be caused by an accumulation of testosterone in the prostate. Within the prostate the enzyme known as 5-alpha reductase converts the male sex hormone, testosterone, into another more potent hormone known as dihydrotestosterone (DHT), the same hormone linked to Male Pattern Baldness. 5-alpha reductase is also present in the skin. Some studies have shown that it may also cause thinning hair in women, as well as producing unwanted body and facial hair growth. DHT controls the division of cells in the prostate. This compound stimulates the prostate cells to multiple excessively, eventually causing the prostate to enlarge.

CHAPTER 3 / The Prostate & Male Pattern Baldness

Normally DHT would be excreted from the prostate gland in sufficient quantity to prevent enlargement. However, if there is an imbalance between the male hormones (androgens) then the DHT is not adequately excreted, causing the prostate to swell. Examination of an enlarged prostate usually reveals three to four times the normal levels of DHT.

The greatest danger that follows Benign Prostatic Hyperplasia is that of a possible malignant change occurring. The metabolites (breakdown products) of cholesterol are cancer producing, and have a tendency to accumulate in the prostate gland. These metabolites initiate a degeneration in the prostate cells which can promote prostatic enlargement.

There is a high correlation between prostate cancer and fat consumption. Worldwide autopsies reveal that wherever the diet is similar to a typical North American one (i.e. high animal fat consumption) nearly twenty-five per cent of all men develop latent cancer of the prostate by the time they reach old age. The Journal of the National Cancer Institute reported that men who ate red meat at least five times a week had a two and a half times greater risk of developing prostate cancer than did men who ate red meat less than once a week (based on a study of 51,000 men).

Countries with the highest prostate cancer death rates are Denmark, The Netherlands, the USA, Canada and the UK. Those with the lowest include: The Philippines, El Salvador, Japan, Columbia, and Mexico.

Diets high in saturated fat and cholesterol have a tendency to clog up the arteries. This reduces and sometimes obstructs blood flow to the heart and brain, not to mention the scalp. Artherosclerosis also tends to reduce blood flow to all the organs, including the reproductive ones, often producing impotence in older men. A study by the Chief of Urology at Metropolitan Hospital in New York found that men with BPH had 80% more cholesterol in their blood than those without the condition.

Maintaining cholesterol levels at a safe limit involves watching fat consumption. But it also must include restricting sugar intake and ensuring an adequate amount of fiber. Both sugar and fiber are involved in the body's ability to process and utilize cholesterol.

Another good reason to include a high-fiber content in your diet is the need for bowel regularity. Constipation is a frequent symptom accompanying BPH. It is quite possible that the long-term increase in pressure creates congestion in the lower pelvic region, where the prostate lies. Not to mention the build-up of bad bacteria that accompanies constipation, which can lead to prostate infection.

The mineral zinc has been shown to inhibit the activity of 5-alpha reductase, the enzyme that aids in the conversion of testosterone to DHT. Unfortunately, the zinc levels in the average man are seldom adequate (see chapter 6: 'Minerals'). And along with this deficiency comes higher 5-alpha reductase levels.

The prostate gland normally contains about ten times more zinc than any other organ in the body. As a preventative supplement fifteen to thirty mg per day is usually sufficient. If one already has an enlarged prostate more research is advised, for this requires a complete supplementation program in conjunction with dietary controls. There are indications that those with BPH also have an imbalance in the quantities of and ratios between their essential fatty acids. Men that showed a high plasma level of alpha linoleic acid had eight times the risk of developing prostate cancer than a control group.

The Townsend Letter for Doctors reported a limited, uncontrolled study in which BPH patients were supplemented with EFAs "...all nineteen subjects showed a diminution of residual urine, with twelve of nineteen having no residual urine by the end of several weeks of treatment."

A familiar face in the war against hair loss shows up in the European research into prostate problems. Nettle Root Extract has been used successfully to exert a decongestive action on the prostate, thus relieving the discomfort resulting from enlargement of this gland. Nettles are rich in vitamins, minerals, and lipids. They have been shown to actually inhibit the

CHAPTER 3 / The Prostate & Male Pattern Baldness

activity of 5-alpha reductase, as well as supporting endocrine gland activity.

Perhaps more substantial than Nettles in the treatment of BPH is the use of Saw Palmetto Berries. A standardized, fat-soluble extract of the fruit of Serenoa Repens (Saw Palmetto Berries) can alleviate the major symptoms of BPH in a surprisingly effective manner. The extract is effective at preventing the conversion of testosterone to DHT, and also inhibits the binding of DHT to cellular and nuclear receptor sites, thereby increasing the breakdown and excretion of DHT.

A suggested dose of Saw Palmetto is 160 MG of standardized extract taken twice per day. Pumpkin seeds, a traditional remedy for prostate problems are not only a high source of zinc, but also contain traces of the hormones normally produced by the prostate. It too inhibits the conversion of testosterone to dihydrotestosterone. Bee pollen also features these three elements, and has been used for BPH.

Currently a human-harvested pollen from rye flowers has been the subject of successful research. It seems to address all three prostate issues: treats BHP, prostatitis (prostate infection) and high PSA levels (a benchmark of cancer potential).

Now that the mechanism of prostate disorders is understood pharmaceutical companies have begun studies of drugs known as 5-alpha reductase inhibitors, which block the action of this enzyme. One such drug, known as Proscar, is marketed by Merck and Co., of Rathway, NJ, as a treatment for non-cancerous prostate enlargement. Saw-Palmetto extract is not only significantly less expensive than Proscar, but has shown a thirty per cent higher success rate in reducing symptoms. Already research has begun with Proscar to determine whether it will be a 'new Minoxidil,' so to speak.

Though it doesn't produce the feminizing characteristics of other anti-androgen medications the results so far have been 'disappointing.'

CHAPTER 4 Dietary Concerns

WHILE IT IS TRUE that hair is essentially dead tissue, hair growth at the root level is a living part of your body. As such, it is as dependent on the nutritional quality of your blood as any other part of your body. If the diet does not contain all the necessary vitamins, minerals, proteins, essential fatty acids and trace elements, the blood will be deficient. Correspondingly, hair growth will be unhealthy and weak.

A variety of nutritional deficiencies have been associated with hair loss, especially those involving the B-complex vitamins. It is well established that severe malnutrition will cause hair loss, and while this extreme is uncommon in the western world, sub-clinical B-complex deficiencies are extremely common.

The refining of whole grains removes a primary source of B vitamins, as does boiling or over-steaming vegetables, since the B's are water soluble. The modern diet is often lacking in raw leafy greens, another major source of many B vitamins. To make matters worse, the vitamins that are ingested are often diverted in order to facilitate the digestion of refined carbohydrates, including sugar, white flour and other refined grains whose own B vitamins have been stripped away in the refining process.

Stimulants such as alcohol, caffeine, nicotine and sugar, have a two-sided effect on the body in relation to hair loss. They rob the body of nutrients they lack as they pass through the system. They also affect the adrenal glands. Long-term use of these substances will leave the adrenal glands in a stressed and depleted state, creating additional nutritional demands on the

CHAPTER 4 / Dietary Concerns

body and, more significantly, raising androgen levels. The lost nutrients and higher levels of male hormones are both of negative consequences for healthy hair.

All steroid hormones produced in humans are made from cholesterol, a substance manufactured within the body by the liver. A high intake of animal foods (especially dairy products like butter and cheese as well as fatty meats) brings an excess of cholesterol into the system. High levels of cholesterol are associated with high levels of DHT, the byproducts of testosterone that is linked to both Male Pattern Baldness and prostate problems.

In 1955 New York scientist Dr. Eugene Foldes followed up on Swedish experiments linking salt intake to hair loss. Dr. Foldes suspected that salt actually accumulated in some tissues, disturbing their function. To test this theory he simply administered a diuretic to a test group. This would cause a body to excrete fluid, and with it excess salt from the tissues. The results were impressive; in some patients hair loss was reduced by as much as 60%.

Reducing the amount of salt in the tissues of the scalp is as simple as reducing salt intake. As the necessary daily requirement for sodium is only 0.2 to 0.6 grams, this is easily obtained in a normal diet without adding any salt at all. A safer alternative to common table salt is true sea salt (commonly referred to as "celtic salt"), which contains a healthier balance of minerals. True sea salt is only 35% sodium, compared to common table salt and refined sea salt, which are 98 to 99% sodium.

Should you wish to experiment with a diuretic, it is strongly recommended that you purchase a herbal diuretic from a health food store, which is a safe and effective alternative to diuretic drugs and their inherent dangers.

When a diet is low in fiber, undigested food remains in the system longer than is necessary. This causes bacterial changes (fermentation) that not only inhibit the quantity and quality of nutrients entering the bloodstream but also allow for the entry of more toxic byproducts. Since the hair follicles are dependent on the quality of nutrients they receive from the blood, a low

CHAPTER 4 / Dietary Concerns

fiber diet will also affect hair growth negatively.

Hair is dominantly comprised of protein, so it follows that one should be assured of an adequate daily protein intake. Protein malnutrition in the western world occurs mostly among strict vegetarians, people on crash diets and those with severely abnormal or poor eating habits. Excessive hair loss begins after two or three months as the body shifts the hair growth cycle into the resting phase in an attempt to conserve protein.

Do not, however, make the mistake of eating too much protein in an attempt to prevent hair loss, as a high-protein diet is detrimental to your general health. Carl Pheiffer of the Brian-Bio Institute, in Princeton, NJ, and Dr. Michael Colgan determined that when protein exceeds 15 to 20% of the diet, the body enters a 'negative mineral balance,' resulting in hair loss akin to that caused by too little protein.

Total protein intake should not exceed about half your bodyweight in pounds converted into grams of protein per day; thus the daily protein requirement of a 180 lb man doing light work is 80 to 90 grams (those in the sports field will disagree, but we are not talking about athletes here). Remember, most of the men in China, India, Japan and Mexico have handsome, thick hair throughout their lives, yet by western standards they live on a very low protein diet. Studies of the nutritional habits of the people in these countries show their diets to be rich in the nutritive elements necessary for hair growth.

The Chinese eat a great variety of vegetables, which they do not overcook. Their diet is rich in rice, soybeans, and high-protein/low cholesterol seafood. Chinese cuisine is high in the vitamins, minerals and essential fatty acids important for healthy hair. Traditional Japanese diets incorporate plenty of seafood and seaweeds, which are rich in Iodine, one of the most important nutrients for hair health. In Mexico and India, rice and beans is the dietary staple, and the consumption of fresh whole fruits and vegetables is the norm.

Another important dietary concern is nutritional mal-absorption. A nutri-

CHAPTER 4 / Dietary Concerns

tious diet is practically worthless if the body is unable to absorb the elements it requires. As our body ages our production of stomach acid decreases. This weakness shows up first in the digestion of protein. The more obvious signs of poor digestion are gas, heartburn and bloating. A feeling of exhaustion following a meal could indicate that too much energy is being spent in digestion.

The digestive process involves several different stages. The first begins in the mouth, where chewing helps convert solid food to a liquid medium. Saliva initiates the digestive process, breaking down carbohydrates and preparing foods for the digestive tract. Chewing triggers the secretion of stomach acids and initiates peristalsis (the movement of food through the digestive tract). If these signals are not received, a heavy burden is placed on the digestive system.

The next level of digestion occurs in the upper-stomach. A variety of enzymes begin to break down the food. The pancreas both stores and produces these enzymes. Enzymes are stored when raw food is eaten, and are used up in the digestion of cooked food. The typical North American diet, which overemphasizes cooked and processed foods, will produce a pancreas that by middle age is unable to produce adequate amounts of enzymes. This may be treated therapeutically with a full-spectrum enzyme complex, available in health foods stores.

However, chronic use of such products, as well as 100% raw foods diets, will weaken the pancreas by making it "lazy" and can lead to dependence. A more permanent solution involves changing the ratio of raw to cooked foods consumed. The pancreas can also be stimulated to produce its own enzymes with herbal combinations and lactic acid products ("Molkosan," miso and sauerkraut).

The third stage of digestion occurs when hydrochloric acid is secreted for further breakdown of food. Insufficient stomach acid is a common problem that can, unexpectedly, result in heartburn, something usually associated with excessive acid levels in the stomach. The excessive use of antacids can worsen digestive disturbances in the long run. An easy way to determine whether or not an imbalance exists is to take a tablespoon of apple cider vinegar or lemon juice (in a little water) at the onset of heartburn. If symptoms clear up, you are deficient in stomach acids; if they are aggravated, stomach acid is excessive. Apple cider vinegar is an inexpensive and effective digestive aid for those with hydrochloric acid deficiency. Five minutes before a meal mix a third of teaspoon with one teaspoon water, swirl it your mouth, and swallow.

After passing through the stomach food is almost entirely digested. It enters the intestines, where the "friendly" bacteria commonly known as acidophilus become involved. Acidophilus is the dominant bacteria in a healthy gut. Its digestion-related functions include a role in enzyme production and the transportation of vitamins and minerals into the bloodstream.

Other functions include immune system support, colon cancer prevention, control of cholesterol levels and the regulation of hormonal fluctuations. Acidophilus bacteria are destroyed by many aspects of modern living, including smoking, chlorinated tap water, rancid oils and food poisoning.

Antibiotics are by far the most destructive, for they do not discriminate between the good and bad bacteria in the body. Low levels of acidophilus can lead to high levels of undesirable bacteria associated with numerous health problems including candida yeast overgrowth. Without active supplementation the digestive system will never fully recover the beneficial bacteria lost after a round of antibiotics.

Symptoms of a lack of friendly bacteria include gas and flatulence, bad breath, pimples and blemishes, bloating, indigestion and headaches. While most traditional diets contain a cultured food rich in friendly bacteria (eg. Yogurt, sauerkraut, sourdough, miso), they serve a maintenance purpose only. These foods are not sufficient to counteract antibiotics, nor can they serve a therapeutic, restorative function.

Therapeutic acidophilus is best suited to this purpose. It can be purchased in a concentrated, encapsulated form in the refrigerator section of most health food stores. It should ideally be taken on an empty stomach with

CHAPTER 4 / Dietary Concerns

water, in order to bypass harsh stomach acids so that it may implant and colonize in the intestines. Acidophilus may be taken after a meal to alleviate heartburn caused by excessive stomach acid. In this case the best form to use would be one in a calcium base.

There is a dangerous tendency in the standard American diet to create a buildup of fat and mucus deposits along the intestinal walls. This layering is the result of a high fat, high protein diet combined with low fiber levels. This condition prevents nutrients from passing through the intestinal wall into the bloodstream. Nutritional deprivation is the result, and it becomes increasingly difficult to feel satiated by a meal.

The safest and easiest way to eliminate this buildup is to add a fiber agent to the diet. This will also keep cholesterol levels down and prevent congestion in the prostate area. Psyllium husks, commercially available in bulk or in fiber formulas are commonly used for this task, unfortunately 'The Safe Shopper's Bible' indicates that psyllium from India is contaminated with both Lindane and Benzene Hexachloride, both dangerous pesticides. At this point it appears that all commercially available psyllium comes from India.

An alternative to psyllium, for those not getting enough fiber in their diet, is to grind flax seeds in a coffee grinder and add a few tablespoons (uncooked) to your oatmeal, protein shake or (sugar-free) granola. Ideally, the ground seeds should be allowed to sit and absorb liquid for 15 minutes to half an hour before eating, but this is not critical.

Grinding the flax not only helps with regularity, but also ensures the anti-cancer benefits of the flax fiber ('lignans') are combined with the breast and prostate protective effects of the omega 3 essential fatty acids found in the flax oil. Avoid grinding more than a 3-day supply of flaxseed, as it is very prone to going rancid, which then makes it toxic.

To maintain freshness, the ground flax should be stored in the fridge in an airtight container. An easier option is to buy defatted flax powder and flax oil, both of which are stable on their own, and convenient to use.

CHAPTER 5 Vitamins

IT IS, OF COURSE, NECESSARY that all nutrients be provided to the body in sufficient amounts for one to attain and maintain good health. The quality and quantity of one's hair is a reflection of that health. However, it is beyond the scope of this book to be a primer on the proper levels of all required nutrients necessary for general well being.

Therefore, in this section, and the following ones on minerals and other supplements, we shall focus only on those nutrients and substances with a track record of being useful in maintaining healthy hair, preventing hair loss, and regenerating hair growth. The nutritional needs and tolerances of an individual will vary according to body size, metabolism and metabolic type, age, diet, genetics, etc.

We advise you seek more information, either through books, a nutritional consultant, or in discussions at your local vitamin shop, before deciding to take large quantities of any of the substances mentioned. While foodstuffs containing high levels of vitamins and minerals are safe to experiment with, isolated nutrients require more careful thought.

Vitamin A is a basic for maintaining healthy bones, eyes, glands, hair, skin and teeth. In conjunction with silica and zinc, it helps prevent drying and clogging of the sebaceous glands. A deficiency of vitamin A can lead to dandruff and dry, dull hair. Such a deficiency also causes the scalp to thicken, trapping oil and perspiration beneath the surface. In order for the thyroid gland to take in enough iodine (its' major nutrient) to function properly, there must be a sufficient amount of Vitamin A. Iodine is essential for healthy hair.

CHAPTER 5 / Vitamins

Vitamin A deficiency can also lead to a degeneration of the pituitary gland. The pituitary gland controls the structure and output of the thyroid gland by means of a thyroid-stimulating hormone. The thyroid hormone acts as a sort of carburetor to regulate both cell metabolism and the use of nutrients (aided by oxygen) utilized to generate heat and energy.

The most common symptoms of hypothyroidism (low thyroid function) are chronic fatigue, cold hands or feet, pale skin, nervousness, brittle nails and poor memory. Of particular interest are the symptoms of dry, coarse skin and hair, and hair loss. To test yourself for an under active thyroid simply keep a thermometer by your bed. In the morning place the thermometer under your arm for fifteen minutes. Keep very still, as the slightest movement can affect body temperature. A temperature of 97.6 degrees F or lower may indicate an under-active thyroid.

Of the Vitamin A destroyers in modern life the most dramatic are air pollution (including smoking), overly bright lighting, aspirin, barbiturates, antibiotics, laxatives, and some cholesterol lowering drugs. One good indicator of Vitamin A deficiency is a tendency to squint in the sunlight. If you feel you are especially at risk take Vitamin A in pill form. Most adults can safely consume 10,000 i.u. per day as a maintenance dosage. Seek advice before taking higher doses though, as Vitamin A is a fat soluble nutrient, and as such is stored by the body, unlike water-soluble nutrients (including the B-vitamins) which wash through the body each day.

In some instances a high dose of Vitamin A can produce undesirable side effects, such as dry skin and inflamed hair follicles, and so it is important to pay attention to your body while taking such a dosage. Vitamin A rich foods include: Alfalfa, apricots, beets, broccoli, cantaloupe, carrots, Swiss chard, fish liver oils, animal livers, kale, parsley, red peppers, sweet potatoes, spinach, yellow squash, and watercress. Most green or yellow fruits and vegetables are high in Vitamin A.

Biotin, a member of the Vitamin B complex, has shown some success at slowing hair loss. Deficiencies in the B vitamins, such as Biotin, are quite common, and the symptoms are wide ranging. They include: poor appetite,

CHAPTER 5 / Vitamins

lack of energy, sleeplessness, dry skin, dermatitis, graying and/or falling hair, and a disturbed nervous system. Biotin is also valuable for its' high sulfur content. Sulfur is one of the main cleansing agents in our bodies, as well as an element necessary for healthy hair growth (see chapt:6 Minerals).

Biotin works synergistically with vitamin B-2, B-6, B-3, and A. It serves the function of a coenzyme, assisting in cell growth, fatty acid production, the metabolizing of carbohydrates, fats, and proteins, and the utilization of the B-Vitamins. Its' antagonists include raw egg whites, antibiotics, alcohol, sulfa drugs, and rancid fats.

Standard supplemental dosages are in the range of 300 mcg, (this is micrograms, not milligrams) though for therapeutic purposes people take three times as much per day. Remember, isolated B-vitamins required a B-Complex backup. This is required to facilitate their own absorption, and to prevent high levels of one B robbing the body of another. Some rich sources of biotin include egg yolk, brown rice, cauliflower, mushrooms, salt-water fish, soybeans, poultry, and nutritional yeast.

One exciting study done with Biotin took the approach of using it externally. In a series of tests involving balding men, Biotin was used instead of estrogen (commonly used in scientific experiments to counteract testosterone, believed to be responsible for male pattern baldness) in a penetrating cream applied to the scalp daily.

The cream having a Biotin-content between .25 and 1% also contained Niacin, a histamine releasing form of vitamin B-3. The Niacin was included to stimulate cell growth and reproduction as well as to increase circulation. In addition to the cream the men used a special shampoo used to reduce hair breakage, which included the amino acids L-cysteine and L-menthionine, two of the most important components in the protein that comprises hair.

Unlike the estrogen cream there were absolutely no side effects to the Biotin program. Of the nearly twelve hundred men in the study (ranging in

CHAPTER 5 / Vitamins

age from fifteen to sixty-nine) eighty-nine per cent showed a definite reduction in hair fallout over a six to eight week period. Daily hair loss fell from one hundred to three hundred and fifty hairs per day, down to an average of less than fifty. Preliminary data (the study was incomplete at the time it was published) indicated that an unspecified amount of re-growth occurred in about fifty to seventy-five per cent of the subjects, with the best results occurring among the younger men involved. There is currently on the market a biotin-based lotion, backed up with a shampoo and conditioner, all similar to those used in the above-mentioned study.

Inositol, another part of the Vitamin B-complex family, is a cell membrane stabilizer and antioxidant that has a protective effect on the hair follicles, perhaps by shielding them from membrane damage caused by oxidized cholesterol in the scalp. One of the most important functions of Inositol is to combine with Choline to form lecithin, which metabolizes fats and cholesterol. This not only wards off coronary disease, but by preventing the hardening and narrowing of the arteries it also helps to keep a healthy blood and nutrient flow to the scalp and hair roots.

Inositiol deficiency has been shown to cause hair loss and graying, in various degrees. Other deficiency symptoms include constipation, eczema, and abnormalities of the eyes. Inositol has a somewhat sedative like effect, and so is beneficial for insomnia, and can relieve mild hypertension through gradually lowering blood pressure. Clearly, this is a supplement to be considered where stress is playing a major role in hair loss. Excessive caffeine intake will rob the body of Inositol, therefore heavy coffee and black tea drinkers should consider supplementation.

Amounts recommended range from 100 mg to 200 mg per day. Inositol is found naturally in unprocessed whole grains, citrus fruits, nutritional yeasts, unrefined molasses, legumes and lecithin.

Niacin is the form of Vitamin B-3 often used as a cholesterol- lowering agent. However, the dosages required to do this (up to 2000 mg per day) were becoming questionable due to the possibility of liver damage. This damage seemed to only occur when timed-release Niacin was used, and now the 'flush-free' form of Niacin is used, which is totally safe. For our purposes, including the circulatory benefits, we will use the flushing kind of niacin, as it is superior for improving circulation to the extremities. There is little or no danger, as one need only 'flush' lightly, and this requires only a small dosage of Niacin. Begin with 25 mg, taken with a meal. Increase dosage until a superficial red rash appears on the skin along with a distinct tingling sensation.

This is caused by the release of histamine, which will flush blood to the extremes of the capillaries, to obvious circulatory benefit. Most people flush at around the level of 100 mg. One may increase the dosage gradually once you build a tolerance to this level, and no longer flush. After a few weeks of this you will notice that the rash has taken on the appearance of an even sunburn, indicating that the once closed capillaries have opened up to receive blood flow.

Should the reaction be too unpleasant, take Vitamin C or aspirin, both of which are anti-histamines. You will literally feel increased blood flow to the scalp. Choose a time to ingest the Niacin when you will be home for awhile, since about 20 minutes after ingesting the niacin the flush will come on and your skin will remain a bright red for about 15 or 20 minutes more.

Do not confuse niacin, a vasodilator, with the other form of B-3, Niacinamide, which is used therapeutically for other purposes. Niacinamide will not cause flushing nor histamine release, and serves no function for reversing hair loss. Aside from the wonders Niacin performs on circulation, a dominant metabolite of the histamine it releases is Heparin, perhaps the most important mucopolysaccharide involved in hair growth.

Mucopolysaccharides work with Collagen as the biological cement that holds tissues together. As mentioned above, histamine release is essential for cell growth and reproduction. As it is only possible to receive the histamine releasing effects from Niacin as an oral supplement we shall dispense with mentioning those foods high in B-3.

CHAPTER 5 / Vitamins

PABA (Para-aminobenzoic acid) is another member of the B Vitamin family. Much like Inositol it is an antioxidant and a membrane stabilizer. Acting as a coenzyme, PABA participates in the breakdown and utilization of protein, and assists in the formation of red blood cells. PABA has shown some success at retarding hair loss and reversing premature graying caused by stress or nutritional deficiency.

In 'Diseases of Metabolism' Dr. F.A. Evans revealed that: "...falling hair was reported by some obese women, after several months on an extremely restricted diet (350 to 450 calories per day)."

These were diets high in protein and not believed to be grossly deficient in any nutrients, yet the women in question lost large amounts of hair. When PABA was supplemented hair growth returned. In a related small scale study, daily doses of 1000 to 3000 mg of PABA gave a response similar to that of Inositol: a reduction of hair loss, but no new growth, and in some cases a darkening of graying hair.

As a part of total dietary regimen PABA is usually recommended in doses of around 100 mg per day. Sulfa drugs may rob the body of PABA. The best sources of it are mushrooms, cabbage, sunflower seeds, oats, spinach, eggs, whole grains, and nutritional yeast.

Pantothenic acid (B-5), often referred to as the Anti-Stress Vitamin, plays a key role in the production of the adrenal hormones and is involved in the formation of antibodies. It aids in the utilization of other vitamins and helps to metabolize fats, carbohydrates, and proteins. Bulb and follicle atrophy, hair loss and graying are B-5 deficiency symptoms, as are adrenal exhaustion, hypoglycemia, fatigue, irritability, nervous system disorder, skin problems and premature aging.

Pantothenic Acid has been able to increase the life span of laboratory animals by over twenty per cent, and at the same time produced increased stamina and endurance. It has also proven helpful in treating anxiety and depression. Recommended dosages range from 100 mg three times a day for hair loss programs, to a total of 1000 mg per day for other disorders. The richest food source of B-5 is Royal Jelly, a product harvested from bees. This is perhaps the main reason why Royal Jelly is touted as a longevity substance and is so popular for a wide range of ailments, including fatigue. Royal Jelly also contains every essential nutrient considered necessary to support human life. Other food sources of B-5 include eggs, beans, nuts, salt-water fish, fresh vegetables, bee pollen, and nutritional yeast.

As a group, the B-Vitamins are of particular value in helping to counteract the harmful effects of high stress levels. Members of the Vitamin B-complex group that play a supportive role in hair and follicle health include B-2, B-6, and Folic Acid.

The B's, however, are interdependent; they require one another for proper body assimilation. Because they never exist in isolation naturally it is best to take a B-Complex supplement, in addition to any particular ones you may wish to focus on. As with most vitamins (and minerals) high levels of B's are most effective when taken in divided doses, with food, throughout the day.

Three times a day is most efficient. In order that the body not become overly dependent on such supplementation, it is a good idea to skip the weekends with all nutritional supplements that are not directly treating an illness.

Bee Pollen, a long time staple of the health food industry, has been mentioned in many anecdotal reports from those suffering from hair loss. After taking Pollen over a long period of time (initially for other reasons) a new strong growth of hair often appeared. Bee Pollen contains 35% protein, half of which is in the form of free amino acids, which can be immediately assimilated by the body. It is also high in Vitamins A, C, D, E, all the B's and lecithin.

A complete 'super-food,' Bee Pollen contains every substance needed to maintain life. This nutritional powerhouse has been used around the world for centuries and is presently very popular with athletes. Being rich in the amino acid L-Cysteine may be one reason why Pollen has a beneficial effect on arresting hair loss and stimulating new growth. The composition

CHAPTER 5 / Vitamins

of hair is approximately 8% L-Cysteine, an amino acid formed from L-Methionine, with an extremely high Sulphur content.

L-Cysteine is utilized as a component of some vitamin compounds on the market that are designed to aid hair growth, but it may also be purchased in its pure form. This may be worth considering since it has a wide range of other important benefits. It helps to detoxify harmful toxins, protects and preserves cells, and promotes fat burning and muscle building. As well as protecting cells from the effects of radiation, it protects the brain and liver from the damaging effects of alcohol and cigarettes.

High doses of L-Cysteine can lead to an increase of Cystine, the oxidized and unstable form of L-Cysteine, unless high doses of Vitamin C are taken. This also helps prevent the formation of Cystine kidney or bladder stones. It is recommended that three times as much Vitamin C as L-Cysteine be taken. Since the average dose taken as part of a hair-rebuilding regimen is 500 mg twice a day, make sure that you take three grams (3000 mg) of Vitamin C in divided doses each day.

A newer version of L-Cysteine, with none of the dangers of stone formation, is N-acetylcysteine. It is also a powerful lung and immune supportive, but should not be used at any level higher than 1000mg per day, without professional advice. Some of the richer food sources of L-Cysteine are eggs, alfalfa, carrot, beet, cabbage, cauliflower, onion, garlic, kale, horseradish, brussels sprouts, legumes, apples, currants, pineapples, hazelnuts, and filberts.

Two other vitamins important to hair growth are C and E. Vitamin C has a multitude of health maintenance functions. It plays a key role in Collagen formation, improves scalp circulation and is required for adrenal gland function, which is necessary to keep stress levels under control. Daily dosage should be in the range of 500 to 3000 mg, in a buffered (i.e. non acidic) form to avoid stomach irritation or diarrhea. A good Vitamin C product should include 'Bioflavonoids,' a co-factor of C, which helps to strengthen veins and capillaries.

Vitamin E also improves circulation to the scalp by increasing oxygen uptake. E deficiency symptoms include hair loss and brittle hair. Supplementation with E can strengthen the heart and immune system. Begin with 400 i.u per day, and work up to 800 i.u. over the course of a few weeks.

Always use natural source Vitamin E (referred to on the label as 'd'alpha tocopherol') rather than the synthetic form derived from petroleum (dl'alpha tocopherol). The synthetic form is not only far less biologically available to the body, but actually blocks E-receptor sites, making it difficult for the body to assimilate Vitamin E in the future. When choosing a Vitamin E product, pick one that is a 'mixed' vitamin E.

Supplementation with Vitamin E can be contraindicated in case of high blood pressure. As is the case with all isolated nutrients, if you have a serious illness you should consult your physician before beginning supplementation.

An important fact to remember about the assimilation of vitamins is that they and minerals require each other, in sufficient amounts ('co-factors') in order to facilitate their respective absorptions. Therefore, if one is lacking you will not properly absorb the other. The implication here is that you must have a good, well-rounded diet in order to properly utilize these supplements. Just as no single food will guarantee good health, no single, isolated supplement can guarantee healthy hair.

CHAPTER 6 Minerals

SOME YEARS AGO, the sheep farmers in the Great Lakes regions found that they were having difficulty getting their sheep to grow wool. This area, like many others, was known to have Iodine-deficient soil. Therefore the grazing plants were similarly deficient. This type of problem is quite common, and easily remedied. Once Iodine was added to the sheep's rations the quality and quantity of their wool immediately improved. Our general health could also be greatly improved by such rational and direct thinking regarding diet.

Certain mineral deficiencies are so common in our part of the world that the resulting conditions (thyroid problems, prostate cancer, hair loss) are taken as a matter of course, yet preventative measures could be taken quite simply, and produce remarkable results.

Your hair's roots must receive proper mineral nourishment in order to perform the function of growing and maintaining a healthy head of hair. Once denied these nutrients the scalp tissues begin to break down, and hair loss results. While all minerals are required in balanced proportions to promote good health, some of them stand out as key players in the health of your hair.

Iodine deficiency in humans first manifests itself as prematurely gray, dry and stringy hair with lackluster quality, and degrees of hair loss. By regulating the thyroid gland with an adequate amount of Iodine, it issues a steady flow of the hormone Thyroxin and the hair follicles receive the nourishment necessary for healthy growth. Thyroxin works with body proteins

CHAPTER 6 / Minerals

to metabolize and deliver nutrients to the millions of capillary blood vessels, lymph vessels, nerve endings, and sebaceous glands, nourishing and rejuvenating them. The Thyroxin penetrates into the layer of fat beneath the scalp, feeding the hair follicles and prompting the sebaceous glands to secrete sebum.

As a supplement, the Iodine found in seaweeds and ocean plants is most effective. In this form it is naturally balanced with co-factors, and is almost identical to the form found in the thyroid gland. One of the better oceanic sources of Iodine is called Irish Moss, a powerhouse of vitamins and minerals. The rich alkaline nature of Irish Moss helps to maintain the body's delicate acid-alkaline balance, another important factor in regulating the flow of thyroxin from the thyroid gland. Irish Moss also contains Vitamin A, D, E and K, as well as Calcium, Sodium, Phosphorus, Potassium, Sulfur, and Essential Fatty Acids.

The seaweed Kelp is the most commonly recommended and available source of Iodine in supplemental form. It also contains a wide range of vitamins and other minerals, including Biotin, Inositol, PABA, Calcium, Sulfur, and Zinc.

Kelp should be taken in quantities of six to ten tablets per day, for therapeutic purposes. This may seem like a lot to take, but remember that this is a food (a 'super food' if you will) and not a vitamin or mineral pill, which is a concentrated and isolated nutrient (albeit, sometimes combined with other concentrated and isolated nutrients). Iodine supplementation is not advised for those on thyroid medications or synthetic thyroid hormones.

Prior to dramatically increasing your daily intake of organic Iodine with supplementation, it is advisable to first discontinue the use of synthetic Iodine, which is added to all common table salt. Switching to non-iodized sea salt is a good idea. This helps curb the potential for Iodine overload. Synthetic Iodine, because it is not provided with its' natural co-factors, does not assimilate well, and many people consume too much salt to begin with. This synthetic Iodine builds up in the body, often overwhelming the thyroid and inhibiting its' proper function. A trace amount of Iodine is naturally present in unrefined sea salt. While ocean plants are our prime source of Iodine, there are other rich food sources. These include salmon, sardines, seafood, lima beans, molasses, eggs, potatoes (with skin), watercress, and garlic.

According to Denham Harman, MD. professor of medicine and biochemistry at the University of Nebraska, the diets of most American men are deficient in zinc. Zinc deficiency can cause derangement of the hormonal rhythms, including that of the thyroid gland. It is essential for the proper functioning of more than seventy enzyme systems.

Zinc's involvement in hair health stems from its role in protein synthesis, collagen formation, and the maintenance of a healthy immune system. Its dosage in supplemental form ranges from fifteen to fifty mg per day. But caution must be used in self-prescribing zinc. While an insufficient amount will impair the immune system, so will an excess of Zinc. Zinc can also rob the body of Copper, one of its co-factors.

One interesting thing to note about Zinc: when the body is deficient, it cannot be tasted, but when the body is saturated a metallic, acidic and unpleasant taste occurs. Therefore, an easy way to determine your own need is to purchase Zinc lozenges, available where vitamins are sold, and designed to ease sore throats. It's best to get a low potency (about 5 mg) with a minimum of other agents.

By counting the lozenges and taking note of when the taste changes one can, after a few days, roughly determine your body's need for Zinc. Do not take the lozenges on an empty stomach, as Zinc taken this way can cause nausea. Another sign of Zinc deficiency is white spots on the fingernails.

15 mg per day is certainly a safe dose of Zinc for most adults. Because minerals accumulate in the system (they are not water soluble) this amount will safely guard against any depletion, and meet the body's daily requirements. Considering the definite link between Zinc deficiency and prostate problems it is a supplement that most men should be taking. Rich food sources of Zinc include fish and seafood (especially oysters), legumes, egg yolks,

CHAPTER 6 / Minerals

mushrooms, pumpkin seeds, sunflower seeds, soybeans, and nutritional yeasts. Among the richest plant sources of Zinc are oats (which are also very high in Silica, an important trace mineral, mentioned further on.) protein, polyunsaturated fats, fiber, and a good range of vitamins and minerals.

Sulfur has been referred to as nature's "beauty mineral" because of its function in keeping hair glossy and smooth, and the complexion clear and youthful. Sulfur is stored in every cell of the body, with the highest concentrations found in the hair, skin, and nails.

Sulfur is also part of the chemical structure of the amino acids L-Methionine, L-Cysteine, L-Taurine, and L-Glutathione. It disinfects the blood, and helps to protect the body against the harmful effects of radiation and pollution, thereby slowing down the aging process and increasing life span. Sulfur is present in Keratin, the tough protein substance that comprises most of the hair shaft.

Folklore sometimes offers that an onion a day will prevent hair loss, and sure enough, onion is one of the richest food sources of Sulfur. In fact, many researchers believe that the wide range of health benefits attributed to garlic, and now similarly to the onion are largely due to the Sulfur containing nutrients of these foods. Large amounts of Sulfur are also found in dried beans, egg yolks, cabbage, brussels sprouts, fish, and turnips. In order to supplement with Sulfur it is necessary to acquire it as one of the aforementioned single amino acids, and not as part of an amino complex.

Two other minerals to consider briefly are Potassium and Iron. Potassium is involved in regulating the transfer of nutrients to cells, and is required for hormonal secretions. Important to a healthy nervous system and a regular heart rhythm, Potassium aids in proper muscle contraction and works with Sodium to regulate the body's water balance. Potassium levels are depleted and disrupted by diuretic drugs and excess coffee consumption (caffeine is a mild diuretic).

Constant fatigue is one of the symptoms of potassium deficiency. Hair-related symptoms to look for (aside from hair loss) are: lack luster hair, itchy scalp, dandruff, straw-like hair that is unmanageable and mats up, and hair that alternates between extremes of oily and dry. Potassium-rich food sources include avocados, bananas, molasses, dried fruit, nuts, potatoes, yams, and nutritional yeast.

Dry, brittle hair is one of the symptoms of low grade Iron deficiency, as is general fatigue, rough and chapped skin, and ridges that run along the length or breadth of the fingernails. Hair loss itself is a symptom of full-blown anemia. A suspected Iron deficiency is easy to confirm through a blood test obtained from your doctor. If you do decide to supplement with iron, do not use Ferrous Sulfate. This type, most commonly sold in pharmacies is not just constipating, but extremely difficult for the body to utilize. Non-utilized minerals do not wash through the body, but actually accumulate in the system.

In the case of Iron, the accumulation occurs in the liver, potentially leading to liver problems. One should purchase Iron (and indeed all supplements) from a reliable source. Good food sources include green leafy vegetables, eggs, fish, poultry, whole grains, almonds, beets, molasses, kidney and lima beans, dried prunes, dates, raisins, and meat.

Our final mineral, Silica, is one that we shall devote abundant space to, as it is perhaps the most dramatic of all at stemming hair loss. It is important to note that we are talking about hair loss of a particular kind. We must differentiate between hair loss, per se, and what amounts to hair breakage. Have a look at some of the hairs on your pillow in the morning, or in your hairbrush. Hair that is falling out will have a tiny white bulb at the end of it. Broken hair will not.

The white bulb is not the hair root, but is the part of the hair nearest the root with some shed scalp skin or follicle lining attached. Since the root can't come out the possibility for re-growth always exists. In the case of breakage, supplementation with Silica is the most effective means of rebuilding and strengthening the hair. Of course, in most cases the hair loss is a combination of both falling and breakage. However, the elimination of breakage is often half the battle, and the easiest part to accomplish.

CHAPTER 6 / Minerals

Silicon is the second most abundant element in the earth's crust (oxygen being the first), where it is found mainly in the form of Silica, or $SiO2$. Silica is found in the stalks of grains and grasses, and is what gives these plants the ability to stand up against the wind. Some studies from the Soviet Union revealed a slowing of hair loss with Silica supplementation, noting that male skin with a weak growth of hair usually proved to have less Silica than male skin with a strong hair growth.

Silica stimulates cell metabolism and formation, inhibiting the aging process. We use it to maintain and repair our nails, hair, skin, teeth, eyes, and cell walls. The pancreas, thymus, thyroid, and coronary arteries are all rich in silica. It increases bone calcium absorption, as well as collagen levels, making the bones harder and more flexible. This can occur even in the elderly, and in women past menopause, though it is commonly believed that it is not possible for these groups to rebuild bone.

The Silicon content of mucopolysaccharides is extremely high. As mentioned in the previous chapter mucopolysaccharides are natural substances produced by the body that work with collagen as a tissue connector, so all connective and elastic tissues in their healthy state are rich in Silica. However, as the level of Silica decrease with age, these tissues degenerate correspondingly.

Declining Silica contents in human aortic tissues correlate very closely with a decline in the elasticity in the of the aortic vessel wall. It is not unusual for artherosclerotic ('hardened') arteries to contain as much as fourteen times less Silica than healthy arteries.

Because most of our foods are either over-processed or have been grown in soils subjected to demineralization (due to top soil erosion and continued use of incomplete chemical fertilizers) most of the foods we eat are Silica-deficient. One of the richest and best-researched sources of Silica accessible to humans lies in the herb horsetail. The premium supplements to use are prepared through an aqueous, or water extract method from this herb. Never take supplemental Silica that is made from unprocessed horsetail.

CHAPTER 6 / Minerals

Ingesting it straight, ground and tabulated, or encapsulated can have toxic side effects. This can destroy Vitamin B-1 in the body and seriously irritate the digestive tract.

One herbal text reports that aqueous horsetail extract also helps reduce BPH, or inflammation of the prostate. Considering the link between Male Pattern Baldness and prostate problems this is another argument for the use of this supplement. Purchase your product in a health food or vitamin store, talk to someone who understands the difference, and make sure the label refers to 'organic vegetal silica from aqueous extract.' Other commonly used forms of Silica are derived from bamboo, or derived from quartz crystals (described as a 'colloidal' preparation, it is a solution of particles suspended in water).

There are few supplements that can compare to Silica, both for preserving hair and for prolonging general youthfulness of the body. The daily requirement for the average adult is between 10 and 20 mg. The therapeutic dosage (as would be required to quickly retard hair breakage) is two to three times that amount for up to a month, after which one would reduce to a maintenance dose. Rice is particularly high in Silica (remember the Chinese, East Indians, and Japanese, with their healthy hair and rice-based diets?) as are oats. Other food high in Silica include lettuce, parsnips, asparagus, onion, cucumber, strawberry, leek, cabbage, sunflower seeds, Swiss chard, celery, rhubarb, and cauliflower.

Interestingly, soluble Silica can also strengthen the hair externally, perhaps accounting for the time-tested success of Nettle hair lotions. Nettle is another extremely rich source of Silica. Organic vegetal Silica, which is available as a supplement in powder form as well as in capsules, will completely dissolve, so you can easily add it to your regular shampoo. This will stimulate healthier hair growth, strengthen the hair shaft, and assure beautiful shine and luster.

There are one or two Silica containing shampoos currently on the market, but considering the expense of properly isolated Silica one must wonder if there is a sufficient amount in commercial shampoo to accomplish anything

CHAPTER 6 / Minerals

dramatic. To prepare your own concoction simply dissolve two tablespoons of powdered vegetal Silica extract in a few ounces of hot water, then pour into your shampoo bottle and agitate the mixture.

To obtain the optimum amount of minerals from your diet, you should remember that all foods recommended in this, and other sections must be organically grown in order to guarantee the level of nutrients. If a mineral is not in the soil it will not be in the food. Even though a plant may take well over dozens of minerals from the soil modern fertilizing techniques rarely add more than a few back to it (nitrogen, phosphorus, and potassium).

The soil eventually becomes depleted of all other minerals, and the plants no longer supply concentrated levels of these nutrients. Whole grains, seeds, and nuts are the best sources for minerals, along with fresh leafy and root vegetables, fresh fruits and freshly made juices.

These foods should be the basis of your daily fare. In choosing a mineral supplement to cover all the bases, as opposed to focusing on single elements, try to find one as complex and naturally occurring in form as possible. It should contain trace minerals, along with the primary ones ('macro-minerals' such as calcium, magnesium, etc) balanced by nature, not by scientific guesswork.

CHAPTER 7 Essential Fatty Acids

MOST OF US are now aware that vitamins and minerals are essential for the growth and maintenance of a healthy body, but many are unaware of the implications of Essential Fatty Acids (EFAs -previously known as Vitamin F) as an essential third component. EFA deficiency or imbalance is so common that it is present in a majority of diseases including arthritis, attention deficit disorder, cancer, heart disease, and diabetes.

EFAs, which keep the body, mind and emotions operating at a high level of wellness, are referred to as "essential" because they are not produced in the human body. They must therefore be part of the food supply. Some of the recognizable symptoms of low-level deficiency are dry, brittle hair, hair loss, and skin problems ranging from itching and flaking to psoriasis. In more severe cases the symptoms elevate to fatigue, confusion, general weakness, easy bruising, pain, inflammation, and swelling of the joints. In examples of growing animals totally deprived of EFAs, there was in addition to hair loss and eczema, an excessive thickening of the sebaceous glands. This is the strongest link between a lack of EFAs and hair loss.

Two Japanese researchers, Masumi Inaba and Yoshikata Inaba, recently posited the 'Sebaceous Gland Hypothesis.' Their observations revealed that the excess sebum that often accompanies hair loss is the result of an enlargement of the sebaceous gland, which is attached to each hair follicle. The enlarged gland increases sebum production, leading to clogging of the pores and malnutrition of the hair root, as well as raising the level of 5-alpha reductase (See Chapt: 2 Causes of Hair Loss). These researchers, from Inaba Aesthetic Surgery in Tokyo, believe that diet is a more probable

CHAPTER 7 / Essential Fatty Acids

cause of this condition than heredity. They noticed that prior to the introduction of animal fat into their diet after WW2, Japanese hair was thick and healthy, with small sebaceous glands and little scalp oil. It has been noted in western research that thinning hair is often preceded by problems with greasy hair. In conjunction with the fact that EFAs have a normalizing effect on sex hormone response (including both estrogen and testosterone), and the link between these hormones, Benign Prostatic Hyperplasia and Male Pattern Baldness, the argument for EFA supplementation becomes very strong.

EFAs are divided into two main categories: Omega 6's and Omega 3's (Omega 9 is mainly found in olive oil, and based on the benefits associated with the 'Mediterranean Diet,' may be considered a healthful oil). Supplemental sources of Omega 6 fatty acids are Evening Primrose oil and Borage Seed oil. Supplemental sources of Omega 3 fatty acids include flax seed oil (as a liquid) and deep-water fish oils. Eating deep-water fish such as salmon (wild), mackerel, trout, herring or sardines, at least three times per week, can provide a reasonable amount of Omega 3's for the average person.

Prior to 150 years ago, the human diet usually provided an equal ratio of Omega 3 to Omega 6. Now the average North American diet is roughly ten to one in favor of Omega 6. This excess of Omega 6 leads to increased arachidonic acid levels in the body, which cause inflammatory side effects. Inflammation, previously considered to be a benchmark of mainly arthritis, is now linked also to Alzheimer's disease, BHP, cancer, nonbacterial prostatitis and heart disease.

The body's store of Omega 3 fatty acids are depleted by caffeine, alcohol, drugs, pharmaceuticals, smoking, chemical exposure, air pollution and high stress levels. Once we have restored our Omega 3 levels, through avoidance of Omega 6 oils (corn, soy, safflower, sesame, sunflower) and supplementation with Omega 3 oils, then it is safe to go back to consuming Omega 6 oils (in an unhydrogenated, naturally extracted form).

Supplementing with Omega 6 EFAs can be appropriate in circumstances

CHAPTER 7 / Essential Fatty Acids

involving multiple sclerosis, psoriasis, as well as PMS and menopausal problems. The issue becomes more complicated by the fact that even those ingesting lots of Omega 6 oils may not be converting them into Gamma Linoleic Acid (GLA), which is the end product the body requires. Thus one can be put in the position of avoiding Omega 6 containing oils, while consuming GLA products (Evening Primrose oil and Borage Seed oil). If you have any of the above mentioned conditions it is best to talk to a professional in order to determine which oils you require, and how much. The recommended daily dosage of EPO is 1500mg and therapeutic is twice that. Borage oil is twice as strong as EPO in GLA, and so requires only half as much for supplementation.

Of these two types of EFAs, the Omega 3 fatty acids have the most support in the scientific literature, especially for prostate health and also for immune support and the prevention of cancer and heart disease. Most people can safely supplement with the Omega 3 fatty acids. The most common forms used are flax oil and fish oil.

However, since a tablespoon of flax oil (and one requires one to two tablespoons per day), or any oil for that matter, is equal to 14 grams of fat, and since flax oil capsules contain at most 1 gram, you would have to consume at least 14 of them to be in the right ball park. Fish-body oil capsules are much more effective at capsule strength, being 4 to 5 times stronger than flax oil.

This is due to biochemical differences between the plant and the animal forms of Omega 3 fatty acids, much akin to the differences between simple Omega 6 containing vegetable oils and the pre-formed end product, GLA. Some people find fish oil capsules hard to digest, so they are best taken with a large meal that includes fat and protein, or taken as a liquid. Liquid fish oils are used at half to one teaspoon per day. Good quality fish oil products are either distilled in such a manner that leaves no contaminants, or are thoroughly tested for heavy metals and other toxins.

Flax seed oil, by the tablespoon, can be just as therapeutic as fish body oils (which is what almost all scientific studies on Omega 3's have used), if one

CHAPTER 7 / Essential Fatty Acids

reduces the intake of all other Omega 6 oils to a minimum. This basically means avoiding restaurant and fast foods, commercial salad dressings, and eliminating all other oils from the diet except extra-virgin olive oil, high-oleic safflower oil, macadamia nut oil and butter. Remember that you must not cook with flax seed oil, or its valuable properties will be destroyed. Coconut oil is an ideal choice for high-temperature cooking.

Excess saturated fat and trans-fatty acids in the diet, compete with EFAs and actually exacerbates the effect of an EFA deficiency, so avoid taking fatty acid supplements with a meal high in such fats (mostly large amounts of red meat, and deep fried foods). But, do take EFA supplements in capsule form at a meal that includes some fats, to improve digestion and assimilation of these good fats. Other factors that interfere with the body's utilization of EFAs include old age, diabetes, excessive alcohol, nutritional deficiencies, high cholesterol levels, persistent viral infections and the consumption of trans-fatty acids.

Trans-fatty acids are formed by 'bad oils' -that is, vegetable oils which have been hydrogenated (to remain solid at room temperature, e.g. margarine), allowed to become rancid, or heated to high temperatures repeatedly (as in the case of deep fried foods and chips). In modern times good oils were, until recently, almost impossible to come by, outside of fish consumption, and bad oils were consumed excessively. This combination of too many bad fats and too little good fats over decades has lead to a widespread deficiency of EFAs, and quite likely the prevalence of cancer and heart disease.

It should be noted that trans-fatty acids are also responsible for free radical formation in the body. Free radicals are now believed to be also partially responsible for the mechanisms of cancer, heart disease, immune system breakdown and premature aging. Free radicals are combated by anti-oxidants. Some of these are produced in the body; some are ingested in the form of nutrients (the most important being Beta-carotene (only the natural form), Vitamin C, Vitamin E and Selenium).

CHAPTER 8 Juices

THE LITERATURE of the natural foods movement is abundant with information on reducing and reversing hair loss, much of it based on juice recipes. When the health food movement began some decades ago vitamin and mineral supplement pills were not available. Those pioneers in nutritional research and medicine found that the easiest and most effective way to provide the body with high levels of nutrients was to juice organic fruits and vegetables. In this form the specific nutrients of the plant are condensed, requiring little energy in order to be digested. These juices are readily assimilated by the body, and as complex in structure (bound to co-factors) as regular food.

One of the important benefits of juice is its high enzyme content, which helps in digesting the juice itself and is also stored by the body for future use in digesting cooked foods, which lack enzymes. In order to capitalize on the enzyme content, the juice must be made and consumed freshly. The longer a juice is stored the more the nutrients deteriorate, the enzymes going first, the minerals last. Bottled juices will provide minerals and some vitamins, but having been pasteurized to prolong shelf-life, are devoid of enzymes.

Following are the most commonly recommended juices for hair loss problems. Most of the foods mentioned can be used interchangeably in recipes of your own devising. These formulations are all based on vegetable juices. However, should you wish to experiment with fruit juices remember that for optimal digestion and assimilation they should be ingested separately. Based on human digestive cycles, fruit juices are best taken in the morning,

CHAPTER 8 / Juices

and vegetable juices in the afternoon. Of course, all the mineral and vitamin rich foods suggested for juicing may also be incorporated into the daily diet as whole foods, to great benefit.

In the 1950's Dr. H. Kirschner had a reputation for reversing hair loss with his program of mineral supplementation. For the most part the minerals were extracted from freshly squeezed vegetable juices. Based on the principle of furnishing food to the scalp nerves and roots of the hair via the bloodstream, his most frequently used treatment was carrot juice. Organic carrot juice contains most of the minerals required by the body, and is rich in Silica, Sulfur, Iron, and Potassium. It also creates an alkaline balance in the bloodstream, strengthens the nervous system, and works on the endocrine glandular system, to help it issue valuable hormones needed by the hair roots.

Carrot juice is enhanced by the addition of cucumber, which due to its high Silica and Sulfur content, is also recommended for the promotion of hair growth. Cucumber also contains Vitamins A, B-Complex, and C, as well as Calcium, Manganese, Phosphorus, Potassium, and Sodium. Naturally occurring sodium as a balanced constituent of food should be of no worry to anyone, and will not adversely affect blood pressure.

Damaging levels of sodium come from table salt, processed foods, and excess meat consumption. In fact, the sodium content of both cucumber and lettuce, also frequently recommended, actually assists in maintaining the calcium in the vegetable, keeping it in constant solution until it is utilized by the body. Lettuce is also rich in Silica and Vitamin A.

Spinach juice is frequently advised, both in combination with lettuce juice, or in lettuce and carrot combination. Those with a history of kidney stones should avoid spinach, as it contains a large of oxalic acid, a substance commonly implicated in the formation of stones. Non-organic spinach, it should be added, is notorious for its high pesticide content.

Alfalfa juice, in combination with lettuce and carrot juice, is a formulation mentioned repeatedly in the literature concerning the growth of new hair,

CHAPTER 8 / Juices

and restoration of its original color. The Arabs, recognizing its superior level of nutrients and corresponding health benefits named it "Al Falfa", meaning the 'Father of All Foods.' Alfalfa's nutrient content is so high because its roots burrow deep into clean, unused earth (as deep as thirty feet), reaching minerals inaccessible to other plants. Alfalfa is rich in vitamins (A, B's, including Biotin, Inositol, and PABA, C, D, E, and K) and minerals (Calcium, Iron Potassium, Phosphorus, Magnesium, Silica, and Sulfur) as well as trace minerals. High in protein and chlorophyll (which helps, detoxify the bloodstream and build red blood cells), alfalfa is also a source of eight enzymes that are known to help metabolize and assimilate nutrients.

It is important to make the distinction here between alfalfa the plant, which is not commercially available as a foodstuff, and alfalfa the sprout, which is. The sprout, unable to send shoots deep into the earth, does not have the same high mineral qualities as the plant, though is rich in enzymes.

Therefore, the accessible means of obtaining alfalfa is to purchase tablets at your health food store. Make sure they come from organic alfalfa. Like Kelp tablets, six to ten per day are necessary to receive any noticeable benefits.

Nettles are also very beneficial when used in juices, for they are extremely high in Silica, Iron, and Potassium, and also rich in Iodine, Sulfur, and Vitamin A and C. While fresh nettles may be difficult to come by, the dried product is easily purchased, and may be brewed as a tea for daily intake.

Since the time of the Roman Empire watercress was believed effective at reversing falling hair. We now know that healthy hair growth is partially dependent on the Sulfur bearing amino acids. Watercress contains more Sulfur than any other vegetable, excluding horseradish. It also contains Vitamins A and C, B-1, Folic Acid, Biotin, B-3, Pantothenic Acid, and the minerals Potassium, Calcium Sodium, Iron, and Zinc. It is one of the best sources of Iodine.

The juice of the watercress is much too strong to take alone, so try a hand-

CHAPTER 8 / Juices

ful of it along with four or five carrots, half a handful of parsley, a couple stalks of celery, and perhaps some lettuce. Spinach is overpoweringly strong in combination with watercress. Another strongly flavored juice, to be added judiciously, is parsnip, which contains the winning combination of Sulfur and Silica in high amounts, along with Potassium and Phosphorus. Adding a quarter inch thick slice of raw ginger root to four or five juiced carrots, along with a few other choice vegetables, will give both the juice and your circulation some zing.

CHAPTER 9 Circulation

MAINTAINING A HEALTHY HEAD OF HAIR depends in part on the quality and quantity of circulation to the hair roots. If the blood, lymph, oxygen and nutrient supply to any given hair follicle is cut off it will die. Whatever the cause, this is the process that begins hair loss and leads to baldness. The most common and easily remedied cause is tension.

Excess stress affects our minds and bodies. It tightens muscles, causes skin problems such as eczema, and reduces blood flow to the extremities. As a result of the muscular contraction, which accompanies tension, tightened blood vessels constrict the capillaries feeding hair follicles and the hair roots become starved. Stress-induced loss of circulation can work in conjunction with a stressed hormonal system (specifically the androgenic hormones produced by stressed adrenal glands), to create a scalp that is prone to severe hair loss. Due to thinner scalp tissue, men are more prone to baldness as a result of stress than are women.

Another cause of reduced circulation is seborrhea of the scalp. This disorder of the oil secreting sebaceous glands is akin to a common form of dandruff that involves the formation of greasy or crusty scales on the scalp. The most common form of dandruff is the dry, flaky type, and is not linked to hair loss. In both these cases excess sebum (oily secretion) combines with dead cell flakes from normal sloughing, clogging the follicles and inhibiting the hair reproduction cycle. Dry hair will often accompany this syndrome because the oily flakes clogging the follicles prevent oil from travelling down the hair shaft. When sebum combines with excessive scalp perspiration it can form hard, crystalline follicle plugs. This causes follicle

CHAPTER 9 / Circulation

congestion and tissue hardening which inhibit nutrient flow to the hair. Apple cider vinegar and jojoba oil can be especially helpful with these types of problems (see chapt: 10 'Herbs & Plants: External Use').

Arthritis or tightness in the neck and spine can tighten blood vessels in the head, reducing circulation and blood flow. Body massage is an excellent way of relieving tension and tightness. Physical activity will also reduce stress and increase blood flow to the extremities, including the head and scalp. Common sense dictates that we must not only reduce circulatory inhibitors and increase general circulation, but must also dramatically increase blood flow to the very top of the head. There are several effective methods of accomplishing this.

For those who like devices, both the 'Back Swing' and 'Gravity Inversion Boots' (used to hang upside down) will bring greatly increased blood flow to the scalp. However, the Gravity Boots are only for the very fit, whereas the Back Swing may be used by almost everyone (except those with very high blood pressure, or other serious circulatory disorders). In either case, use should begin very gradually and be increased slowly.

Two low-tech, inexpensive options are the slant board and the headstand. The slant board should be used at a roughly forty-five degree angle, working up to fifteen minutes a day. The headstand, a well-known Yoga practice, is even more effective than the slant board. There are those of the opinion that this is the single most important thing one can do to prevent hair loss and improve the health of the hair. Work up to two to three minutes, twice a day. Those with high blood pressure or with poor physical health should not attempt the headstand technique. Inversion-techniques, with the added bonus of increasing the mental faculties by increasing blood and oxygen flow to the brain, are even more effective when backed up with massage techniques.

Finger massage is very efficient way to improve blood circulation to the scalp. However, because it is essential to keep the blood circulating constantly, massaging once or twice a week will not accomplish much. Ideally, scalp massage should be performed at least twice a day in order to be ben-

CHAPTER 9 / Circulation

eficial. Try to include it as part of your hair-washing regimen as a way of working it into a regular habit. Place all ten fingertips firmly on the head and, without moving the fingers, push the whole scalp in circular motion for a few seconds. Then, moving from front to back, and then back to front, place the fingers in a new position and repeat. Cover the whole scalp, including the temples, forehead, and neck, where you may also use an upward pushing motion. Avoid rubbing the problem area, as this could break hairs at the surface and traumatize the follicles.

Some experts allow for a flat-handed scalp massage, placing the palm of the hand against the scalp and rotating, as an alternative to the finger massage. It will loosen the tightness of the scalp, relaxing without damaging any hair but, while it is easier to do, it is not as effective as the finger technique. An effective scalp massage may also be attained using an electric vibrator. The better models have an attachment designed for scalp massage, and are easy to use offering an effortless massage. At the very least use it twice a day for about five to eight minutes, and use a similar motion to that of the finger massage.

How Hair is Nourished fig 3

The importance of complete nutrition becomes apparent when one realizes that the arteries bring nutrient-rich, oxygenated blood to the hair root, while the veins carry away waste products and carbon dioxide

CHAPTER 9 / Circulation

An Oriental circulatory technique (based on Qi Kung) involves the ancient art of raising and circulating body energies. Place your fingers at the center of the base of your skull and bring them to each ear, tapping them gently about thirty times. Repeat this exercise about eight times, beginning a little higher on the skull each time until you reach the crown of your head. This is designed to bring blood to the scalp and face, nourishing the hair and giving the skin a youthful glow.

CHAPTER 10 # Herbs and Plants: External Use

CERTAIN NATIVE AMERICAN TRIBES had a remedy for graying or falling hair that involved the common grape vine (following its' introduction by Europeans). In the spring they would cut off the end of a branch, tie a gourd onto it and collect the sap. The sap was then applied generously and worked into the scalp and roots of the hair. An alternative method was to make a tea of the roots of the grape vine.

This was used as a wash two or three times a month when graying or falling first became apparent, and then used only once a month, once the problem was under control (Interestingly, grape seed extract is currently being studied as a topical application to encourage new hair growth, and has had success in mouse studies).

Few of us today would go to such effort. Yet every culture has had its' own approach to the problem of hair loss, based both on the variety of indigenous plants available and its' cultural perspective. Let's look at a few of the more improbable ancient techniques before approaching those with a stronger historical and scientific base.

From the 'De Material Medica' of the famous Greek herbalist of the first century AD, Dioscorides: '...Wild olive oil will not only prevent hair from falling out, but will also prevent it from turning gray...intended to be rubbed into the scalp daily.'

From the 'Ebers Papyrus,' an Egyptian medical document, four thousands years old: (1) 'Mix together the fat of a lion, fat of a hippopotamus, fat of

CHAPTER 10 / Herbs & Plants: External Use

a crocodile, fat of a cat, fat of a serpent, and fat of a Nubian ibex, and rub the mixture on the head.' (2) 'Mix the crushed flax seed with an equal quantity of oil, add water from a well, and rub mixture on the head.'

Aztec remedies: (1) 'Make a poultice of Nettles, serpents, scorpions and millipedes that have been ground up and boiled together.' (2) 'For hair that will not grow, bathe the head with morning water (urine) from a woman who is with child.'

It is easy to laugh at such remedies when we look at them from the modern perspective, but these were thriving and successful civilizations. One out of two of their members did not die of heart disease, nor did one out of four die of cancer, as do members of our own civilization. Perhaps we would do well then, to look a little closer at the remedies and techniques of bygone people and cultures, as well as out our own folklore.

Before leaving these examples let's consider them from a modern perspective: olive oil and flax oil both provide essential fatty acids, recently proven to be necessary for healthy hair growth. To this day, people of Greek or Mediterranean descent apply virgin olive oil to their hair and scalp to improve hair condition.

Nettles are one of the most common herbs used in natural hair loss remedies around the world. Science has recently found some success in reversing hair loss with the topical application of synthetic estrogen; its' natural analog is prevalent in the urine of a pregnant women.

As mentioned, Nettles have been used as a hair growth stimulant for centuries. They are rich in vitamins A and C, and a wide range of minerals including Iodine, Silicon, and Sulfur, all especially good for the hair. The other two herbs frequently mentioned in herbal texts and folklore are Rosemary, both for cleansing the scalp and stimulating the hair root, and Sage, which is claimed to not only stop falling hair, but to strengthen and thicken the hair shaft.

Two remedies that use all three herbs are: (1) Boil together in water, rose-

CHAPTER 10 / Herbs & Plants: External Use

mary, sage, peach leaf, nettle and burdock: strain and use to wash hair daily. (2) Steep one ounce of ground rosemary, two ounces of ground sage, and half an ounce of ground nettles in one pint of ethyl alcohol for a week: strain and add one ounce of olive oil, one ounce of castor oil and one ounce of water. Shake before using as a hair lotion, either before bed or at least fifteen minutes before shampooing.

Apple cider vinegar is frequently mentioned in folk remedies for hair loss. It is reputed to have a normalizing effect on the scalp's oil glands and pH level. More importantly, its' high acidity and powerful enzymes destroy harmful bacteria responsible for several scalp conditions. Disturbances in the scalp's epidermal cell renewal can cause an accumulation of dead cells at the skin's surface.

Excessive oil gland activity causes the scale-like dead cells to become more firmly attached to the scalp and each other. This forms a breeding ground for the harmful bacteria called 'bottle bacillu.' Itching and dandruff ensue, and hair follicles become clogged. Deprived of natural oils, hair begins to break off or fall out.

The benefits of apple cider vinegar can be obtained as follows: Part hair into sections. Apply two tablespoons directly to the scalp with a moistened cotton ball. Allow between fifteen minutes and three hours before shampooing. In acute cases this can be repeated on a daily basis. An after-shampoo rinse, suitable for the whole body, uses one third of a cup of vinegar per quart of rinse water.

An old English herbal text suggests washing the head once a day with strong, warm sage tea, and using diluted apple cider vinegar as a rinse, to check the falling hair and stimulate growth.

Another old herbal recipe involves making a strong decoction by mixing freshly dried nettles, with equal amounts of water and apple cider vinegar, then simmering it down until it resembles the color of coffee. This is rubbed into the scalp once a day (the text also recommends washing the scalp each morning with cold water, a great aid to circulation).

CHAPTER 10 / Herbs & Plants: External Use

One interesting nettle formula for hair loss includes onion: one part Nettle leaves, one part onion, one part seventy per cent alcohol. Soak the leaves and onion in the alcohol for several days, then massage into the scalp before washing the hair, in order to stimulate hair growth. This simple, inexpensive remedy comes from a highly respected source, Dr. A Vogel, a Swiss herbalist known throughout the world. At the time he wrote this, in 1952, there was available on the European market a deodorized onion scalp lotion.

Essential oils distilled from plants and herbs are an effective remedy for a wide range of hair and scalp ailments. They add luster and shine to the hair and increase circulation to the scalp. In addition, these oils are easily absorbed into the lower levels of the skin, where new cells are generated. Because essential oils are too strong to be applied directly to the skin they must be diluted with a carrier-oil. Jojoba and olive oils are particularly well suited to this purpose.

As a general rule, ten to twenty drops of essential oils should be mixed with one ounce of carrier-oil. Massage into the scalp for a minimum of ten to fifteen minutes before shampooing, or leave on over-night and shampoo in the morning. Some of the most commonly used essential oils for hair loss are Cedarwood, Clary Sage, Lavender, Eucalyptus and Rosemary. Clary Sage helps to dissolve sebum deposits; Lavender regulates the acid mantle of the scalp and gives body and shine to the hair shaft; Eucalyptus regulates sebum, reduces inflammation of the scalp, and is a deep-cleaning agent; Rosemary shares much in common with Lavender.

Most of these essential oils also stimulate circulation in the scalp. Another popular oil is Cajuput or Tea Tree Oil, which is especially good for severe dandruff, and is also an effective disinfectant and bactericide.

Researchers in Scotland recently published a study on the use of essential oils to combat stress-related hair loss, in the 'Archives of Dermatology.' Patients with alopeica areata (an autoimmune condition that can cause temporary and/or total hair loss) massaged their scalps daily with a mixture of

CHAPTER 10 / Herbs & Plants: External Use

Cedarwood (cedrus atlantica also known as atlas cedarwood; other varieties may be toxic), Lavender, Rosemary and Thyme essential oils, mixed with carrier oils. The control group used only the carrier oils: jojoba and grape seed oils. Only 15% of the control group showed significant improvement compared to 44% of the subjects using the essential oils, after seven months of usage.

For centuries Mexican and desert Indian tribes have used Jojoba oil (pronounced "ho-ho-ba"), to keep their hair healthy and to relieve skin problems such as dermatitis, eczema, and psoriasis. Jojoba oil resembles the skin's own natural sebum secretions, and so has a remarkable affinity for skin and hair.

A perfect moisturizer for hypoallergenic skin, it is completely absorbed into the skin's deep layers. Jojoba oil removes sebum deposits, which collect around the hair follicles, solidify and cause dandruff, hair loss, and scalp disorders. It also makes the scalp less acidic, and is great for both dry and oily hair, as well as itchy scalp problems. Jojoba contains B vitamins, vitamin E, Silicon, Chromium, Copper, Zinc, and is high in Iodine.

One of the herbal folk remedies to prove itself to modern researchers is the 'Cayenne Pepper Hair Tonic.' A powerful skin irritant, such as cayenne, will bring good blood flow to the scalp and also cause histamine release, which stimulates cell division, encouraging new growth. The tonic recipe is as follows: Mix four ounces of cayenne pepper with one pint of one-hundred-proof vodka (which is 50% alcohol, or pure grain alcohol diluted with twenty per cent distilled water). Let stand for two weeks, shaking the mixture once each day.

Strain through several layers of fine cloth or a nylon stocking until the mixtures is free of pepper. Once or twice a day rub a small amount onto the thinning or balding areas of the scalp. Avoid contact with the eyes. Effects should be noticeable within five weeks.

Another hair growth tonic that stimulates circulation to the scalp, but is simpler to prepare and use, involves juicing a one to two inch piece of gin-

CHAPTER 10 / Herbs & Plants: External Use

ger root (you may find this easier to do if you grate it first). Just massage the juice into your scalp and let it dry for ten or fifteen minutes, then shampoo. This will create a distinct tingling sensation.

Certain Indian tribes of Mexico claim that their thick, healthy hair, resistant to graying and balding, is due in part to their regular use of the gel from the Aloe Vera plant. They rub the gel into the hair and scalp, and leave it on overnight. The next morning it is washed out without the use of any other cleansing product, such as soap or shampoo, as certain properties of the plant produce a low sudsy action. The plant has been used in the past and present for a number of ailments including arthritis, burns, insect bites, cold sores, dry skin, and internally for ulcers and hiatal- hernias.

Aloe Vera was recently studied by the Japanese (now more prone to baldness as they disregard traditional ways and adopt western eating habits) for its' potential to prevent hair loss, and has shown some success at reducing hair loss. Aside from containing an abundance of amino acids, vitamins, and minerals, Aloe Vera also has the ability to balance the skins' pH level. Its proteolytic (protein-digesting) enzymes help to slough off dead skin cells and open pores.

Due to its content of lignins and polysaccharides, it also helps other ingredients to penetrate more easily and deeply into the skin. One key mucopolysaccharide, known as Acemannan, is most highly concentrated in aloe products made from the whole leaf. Acemannan interjects itself into cell membranes, causing an increase in the membrane's fluidity and permeability. This facilitates the outward flow of toxins and the inward flow of nutrients to and from the cell.

The highest quality Aloe Vera products are those which use the whole leaf (as opposed to just the inside of the leaf) and which offer standardized mucopolysaccharide levels. Aloe also works especially well for drawn and painful scalp conditions, with the advantage of remaining unnoticeable even if used throughout the day. From India comes this recipe for a shampoo designed to stimulate hair growth: Combine and mix seventy per cent Aloe Vera gel, twenty per cent wheat germ oil and ten per cent coconut

CHAPTER 10 / Herbs & Plants: External Use

milk. Wet hair, apply the shampoo mixture and massage into scalp. Leave on for five minutes, then rinse.

Above we have detailed the herbs and plants more commonly referred to in the literature on the subject of hair loss. Following are some random elements mentioned only rarely or in isolation. They are included for those using this book as a reference.

Ginseng root, used as lotion in an alcohol base, is mentioned both in Chinese literature, and is a component of 'Formula 101 hair Liniment,' sold in sixteen countries around the world.

Walnut meat is also a component of 'Formula 101' and, next to flax seed oil, is the richest vegetable source of Omega 3 essential fatty acids. From Europe comes this 'Walnut Leaf Hair Loss Lotion.' Cover two heaping teaspoons of finely chopped walnut leaves with one cup of boiling water, cover with a lid and steep for 10 minutes, then strain, and massage into the scalp daily. The same technique done with marshmallow leaves is also recommended as a remedy.

Nicholas Culpepper (1617-1654), the famous English herbalist offered this solution: Use four ounces of crushed ripe peach pits in one pint of vinegar. Apply three times per day. Here we assume he is referring to apple cider vinegar, and that the formulation must be allowed to sit for a week or two, and then is strained.

While many will choose not to go through the trouble of making their own lotions and tonics, both the raw ingredients mentioned in this chapter and hair loss products containing many of these substances, are available in health food stores and herbal shops. At very least, these are ingredients to look for when choosing shampoos, conditioners, tonics and other hair care products.

Various hormonal remedies have been somewhat effective at countering Male Pattern Baldness (a hormonal affliction) however they are not without their limitations. Typically, they are effective at preventing hair loss, but

CHAPTER 10 / Herbs & Plants: External Use

not as effective at re-growth. In addition, topical applications can easily enter the bloodstream, and, as these are hormonal drugs, can upset the body's delicate balance.

The topical application of female hormones to the scalp has displayed some success at inhibiting DHT formation by blocking its' receptors (as does a testosterone compound salve). However, hair re-growth averages only about ten per cent, and in some cases it was more than a year before any noticeable effects were observed.

A safer alternative is 'Wild Yam Cream,' which contains three per cent natural progesterone. Progesterone is a hormone that provides the building block for all steroid hormones. It has the same nucleus as estrogen and performs similar functions.

The cream is sold by naturopaths and in health food stores. It is used to safely and naturally raise a woman's estrogen levels in order to retain and deposit calcium into her bone mass. It also helps in dealing with symptoms of menopause, helping to forgo the need for synthetic estrogen therapy. The cream base contains a delivery system to carry both through the skin and into the blood stream, in order to penetrate sufficiently into the scalp.

Sarsaparilla extract was discovered in 1939, and is sold under its' Latin name, Similax Officianalus. It contains hormonal compounds similar in structure to testosterone, and is often ingested by athletes seeking to raise their testosterone levels. Available in health food and vitamin stores, the extract is in an alcohol base, which is an ideal delivery system for topical application.

More effective at promoting hair re-growth than topical hormone treatment is a substance called Polysorbate 80. Research done at Finland's Helsinki University claimed an eighty per cent success rate in both women and men, with no significant side effects (although there is an increase in hair loss for the first week or two, due to the loosening of hairs in the resting phase). Re-growth was reported in hundreds of men in their fifties and sixties who used Polysorbate 80 every day for a year.

CHAPTER 10 / Herbs & Plants: External Use

Polysorbate 80 is approved by the FDA for use as a shampoo surfactant and as a food additive. As a food additive it is used as an emulsifier: an agent that causes water and fats to mix. It is considered to be of negligible toxicity, and as such is found in everyday products such as mayonnaise, salad dressings, and some liquid detergents. It is also the base of the "Helsinki Formula", and many other commercial hair loss products designed for external use.

Polysorbate 80 is said to work through removing DHT and cholesterol from the scalp, and causing the release of histamine (a cellular growth factor) in the scalp. Scientists using it were able to reverse a degree of early tissue disorganization occurring at the inception of some chemically induced cancers. Thus, it may also affect the control of genetic activities in the hair follicle cells.

Pure Polysorbate 80 is sometimes available in health food stores or can be purchased through the internet. To use it, coat the scalp with a thin film in the balding areas, ten or fifteen minutes before shampooing. It is a viscous substance, so place several drops on various areas of the scalp, then rub the drops in and around vigorously. The scalp should redden and feel slightly warm due to the histamine release.

Pure Polysorbate 80 washes out easily, though if you get it in your eyes it will be mildly irritating, just like any shampoo. If it is going to work for you, you will notice thin, short hairs within two or three months of daily use. After a longer period the hairs should improve in quality and quantity.

CHAPTER 11 **Devices and Gadgets**

A 1989 STUDY at the University of British Columbia indicated much potential for arresting hair loss through electric pulses to the scalp. Dr. Stuart Maddin, a dermatologist with UBC's Adult Hair Clinic, gave thirty men fifteen minutes of electric pulses once a week, through a hair dryer-like device. By the end of the thirty six week study all but one of the subjects had either increased hair growth or reduced unnatural loss.

The study found that 'electrotrichogenesis' could increase the numbers of hairs on balding men's heads by up to sixty-six per cent. Similar electrical treatments are used to heal bone fractures, speed tissue healing, and remove skin ulcers and scar tissue. In this case the device alters the electromagnetic field around the hair follicles, changing the protein synthesis in the cells. Though the treatment has been approved by the Federal Health Protection Branch in Canada, and is being examined by the FDA in the U.S., Dr. Maddin is unsure whether it will ever become a commercially available treatment.

In 1987 two Canadian entrepreneurs approached the hair loss problem from an unusual perspective: hand reflexology. Reflexology, considered akin to a Western version of acupuncture, is based on physically manipulating acupuncture points on the hands and feet, using the practitioner's thumbs and fingers rather than needles. Reflexologist Mildred Carter, in her book on hand reflexology, highly recommends fingernail buffing for follicle stimulation and healthy hair. She refers to testimonials of new growth, color change, and the prevention of graying.

CHAPTER 11 / Devices and Gadgets

At least one disease of the scalp, Alopecia Areta, which can cause complete hair loss, also produces pitted fingernails.

The 'Hair-Tech' was designed to provide an easy method of nail stimulation in the comfort of your home. It weights in at six pounds, and measures twelve by four inches. A limited study was run with the new device. Thirty men between the ages of nineteen and fifty-nine received a ten-minute buffing of their fingernails, once per day.

Within six weeks those experiencing excessive hair loss were noting a dramatic improvement. After approximately three months on the program various claims were made by the subjects: including improved hair condition, new visible growth, natural color returning, looser scalp, and faster growth of finger nails.

While results varied from person to person, every subject reported that they had stopped losing excessive amounts of hair. It should be pointed out this study was done by the 'Hair-Tech' company. Nonetheless, they offer a guarantee that unnatural hair loss will stop within thirty days, otherwise they refund the cost of the product.

Magnetics are currently enjoying resurgence in the Orient and Europe as therapy for a wide range of ailments including arthritis, muscular pain, and inflammatory conditions. One catalogue offers a 'Magnetic Therapy Brush' with 'Induction Bristles' (made from metal) to invigorate the main acupuncture points of the scalp, stimulating blood circulation. It is claimed that daily use will help prevent hair loss, dandruff, and seborrhea, while strengthening hair and promoting new growth. It also claims to relieve neck pain and stiffness.

It is worth noting that finding even three or four reputable 'devices and gadgets' was a difficult task. This area, more than any other in the hair loss field, should be approached with caution. Look for impartial studies rather than 'personal testimonials' and always check your sources. Remember, a firm dietary base is your primary defense against hair loss. Devices and Gadgets should be considered complementary, at best.

CHAPTER 12 Choosing a Shampoo and Conditioner

EXCESSIVE SHAMPOOING, particularly with most commonly used commercial shampoos, can cause the hair to lose minerals such as Calcium, Phosphorus, Iron, and Nitrogen. This is due to the harsh chemicals present in most of these products. Not only will they damage your hair, but they can also pose a threat to general health. Formaldehyde, which is used in shampoo as a preservative, is often disguised as 'Quanternium–15'.

Aside from being carcinogenic at certain levels, it can prove to be an irritant to the skin, eyes and respiratory system. Shampoos may also contain ammonia, coal tar colors, synthetic detergents, ethanol, and artificial fragrances. It's no wonder allergic reactions to these products are common.

It is safest to purchase your shampoo at a natural foods store, or from a professional at a hair salon. Make sure they can address your concerns about excess chemicals. Read the labels, and don't hesitate

to ask questions. Try different shampoos until you find one that you like, then alternate to a different brand every so often. Remember, the shampoo you used in your twenties may not be the best choice to use in your forties.

This is because hair, like skin, becomes drier as we age, producing less of the oil that serves as a protective shield for the hair shaft. Look for mild cleansers such as cocoamide betaine or cocoamido propyl betaine, which are extracted from coconut, or sulfosuccinates, which are derived from wheat germ oil.

CHAPTER 12 / Choosing a Shampoo

Even Sodium Lauryl Sulfate, and other sulfates used in 'natural' shampoos can strip away too much oil from the hair, leaving a film of shampoo residue. Layered shampoo residues, combined with excess sebum and perspiration salts, can cause follicles to plug. Because these sulfate surfactants are made in a process that uses sulfuric acid, they can become unstable, reverting back to sulfuric acid and irritating the skin, scalp and eyes. Protein or Keratin in shampoo will give hair body and bounce.

By coating the hair, protein fills in gaps and pits in the damaged hair shaft, and temporarily repairs split ends by gluing the frayed ends back together. Hydrolyzed soy protein, containing amino propane sulfonic acid can reinforce the hair and, through regulating sebum production, can also stimulate growth.

One key ingredient to look for is Panthenol (pro-Vitamin B-5). Panthenol is used to improve hair strength and elasticity. It works because the molecule is small enough to actually work its way into the hair cortex, where it can bond to the building blocks of hair. Panthenol can strengthen undamaged hair by up to 20%. Damaged hair shows even more dramatic results. Also look for anti-oxidants such as Vitamin A, C, E, and nourishing herb and plant extracts including Aloe Vera, Burdock, Chamomile, Chaparral, Horsetail, Nettles, Rosemary, and Sage.

A properly balanced shampoo has a pH of 5.5 (the acid range is from 0 to 7 pH, and the alkaline range is from 7.1 to 14.0 pH). A properly balanced shampoo, which is slightly acidic, does not coat the hair but leaves it shinier, and is gentle enough to use daily. A 'body' shampoo is mildly alkaline, and though not harsh enough to be damaging, it tends to swell the hair shaft slightly.

Regular use of a conditioner is necessary to maintain healthy hair (unless you have a buzz-cut). A conditioner is best compared to a skin moisturizer. It is especially important for dry hair and hair overexposed to aggravating environmental conditions such as drying wind, heat, sunlight, and chemicals such as chlorine. Chlorine, for example, chemically bonds

CHAPTER 12 / Choosing a Shampoo

to hair, robbing it of moisture and leaving it dull, brittle, and susceptible to breakage. These environmental factors damage the hair shaft, not the follicle. As such, the condition is preventable. Conditioners coat the hair cuticle with a fine film which smoothes it and temporarily rebinds split ends back together, making the hair appear thicker. Conditioners also reduce static and restore softness, shine, and manageability.

One skincare clinic has suggested that poor quality conditioners can cause clogging of the follicles. It is therefore important to keep the conditioner on the hair, but try to avoid getting much of it on the scalp. If you can stand it, a good cold-water rinse will lay the cuticles down on the hair shaft, accomplishing most of what a conditioner is designed to do. You will also get the benefits of extra blood circulation to the scalp.

As with shampoos, look for a minimum of unrecognizable chemicals, and a clearly defined protein. Keratin, or amino acids, should be included among your conditioner's ingredients(again, for filling in cracks and breaks in the hair shaft, and gluing split ends back together). Check the label to ensure the inclusion of natural oils (unless you have excessively oily hair) such as Safflower, Jojoba, and Evening Primrose.

These lubricate hair strands, reduce tangling, and prevent moisture loss. If your hair is oily, then check the label for a natural moisturizer called 'NaPCA'. NaPCA is found naturally occurring in human skin, and is not oil based. If you have extremely damaged hair you may wish to consider using a deep conditioner once a month. These are specialty products and must be left on for a minimum of ten minutes.

One of the best and safest is the neutral 'henna', a natural clay-like substance, in use since the time of the ancient Egyptians. Henna seals the cuticle, protecting hair and making it glossier. Periodic applications add additional protective coatings.

Currently on the market there are shampoos with built in conditioners. These are best avoided. Shampoo and conditioning serve two different functions, and by combining them the effectiveness of each is decreased.

CHAPTER 12 / Choosing a Shampoo

Anti-dandruff shampoos are among the most dangerous of all hair care products, the other leading two being aerosol hair spray and styling mousse. Dandruff shampoos use toxic medications to prevent the scalp from peeling. The most popular agent is selenium sulfide which, taken in excess, has shown to cause degeneration of the liver and other organs.

Dandruff shampoos may also contain toxic creosol and the carcinogenic 'polyvinyl pyrrlidone plastic' (PVP), not to mention the standard chemicals found in most commercial shampoos. While the FDA maintains that the limited amounts of these toxic substances in a shampoo poses no threat, it is important to remember that the skin and scalp are an avenue to the bloodstream, and that most carcinogens are cumulative (that is: it is not how much you absorbed today, it is how much you absorbed over ten years).

One final world about dandruff: many people with serious dandruff problems maintain healthy hair throughout their lives. For those with thinning hair however, a dandruff problem may worsen the condition. Dandruff itself does not cause baldness. It is the result of increased skin cell production (which is caused in part by excess protein intake) combined with excessive oil secretions.

The two most basic steps in dealing with dandruff are massaging the scalp and brushing hair frequently. This dislodges dead cells. Frequent shampooing (with a mild shampoo that won't dry the scalp) also helps to rid the scalp of dead skin scales and oily secretions.

CHAPTER 13 **Washing, Drying & Brushing**

BEFORE ENTERING THE SHOWER or beginning to wash your hair, give it a good brushing, and massage the scalp as well. These steps will loosen the dirt and scalp flakes, activate the oil glands, and encourage circulation. It is important to pre-rinse for at least one full minute before applying shampoo. This begins the removal of loosened debris from the scalp and facilitates better distribution of a smaller amount of shampoo. Using too much shampoo can leave the hair dull, because the more used the more difficult it becomes to completely remove when rinsing. Avoid using excessively hot water. This can actually increase temporary hair loss by softening the scalp and making it easier to pull hairs from their roots.

To apply shampoo, pour the minimum amount necessary onto the palm of your hand, rub your hands together and smooth the shampoo evenly over your hair. Do not pour shampoo directly on your hair as this saturates one spot to excess. Massage the shampoo into the scalp with the tips of the fingers (not the fingernails, which can irritate the scalp), spreading the lather and gently working the whole scalp area. Then rinse with warm water, and continue rinsing longer than you think is necessary. The ideal final rinsing should be with water moving progressively from cool to cold. Cold water will stimulate circulation and shrink the outer layer of the hair, making it smoother, shinier and more manageable. It also makes the hairs stiffer, stronger and locks them more firmly into their roots.

Some people need to wash their hair every day, some only once a week. Most fall in between these two extremes. How often one should shampoo depends on three factors. The first factor is the amount of oil your scalp nat-

CHAPTER 13 / Washing, Drying & Brushing

urally secretes. Signs of excessive scalp oil requiring more frequent shampooing include dull and limp hair, itchy scalp, and greasy or oily looking hair that cling to the scalp. The second factor is your environment. If you live in a city with high levels of air pollution, then you will need to shampoo more frequently than someone living in a place with cleaner air. Finally, the season of the year is also a factor. During the heat of summer your head will perspire more than in cooler weather, and so requires more frequent washing. In cold, dry winter air your natural oil production may reduce to a point where shampooing is more seldom required.

For those who shampoo once every day, assuming that no unusual amounts of dirt and debris have been picked up, one washing should be sufficient. If those who shampoo less frequently choose to lather-up twice, it is recommended that they use a very mild shampoo. Buy one based on advice from a professional, either at a salon or a natural foods store. Labels can be misleading. A good shampoo will allow for deep cleaning without stripping the hair of its natural oils. When hair is 'squeaky-clean,' it is probably over-cleaned. This is unnecessary and damaging to hair.

After the hair has been washed and thoroughly rinsed, apply the conditioner. Apply in a manner similar to that for the shampoo: pour a little into one palm, then rub the hands together and smooth it over the hair. However, remember that a conditioner is for the hair and not the scalp, so you need not work it into the scalp as you would with shampoo. Conditioners can be used as often as you shampoo, but don't use too much; you can over condition your hair. Excess conditionings can weigh the hair down and reduce, instead of enhancing, luster and body. One with very fine hair may find that frequent use, or certain brands, may cause their hair to have a flat and limp look.

Those with oily hair may find certain brands exacerbate the problem. The answer, as with shampoos, is trial and error. If your hair is not damaged you may opt to use a conditioner only once or twice a week. In any case most conditioners will have done their job within 30 seconds of application, so it is not really necessary to leave it on much longer than that.

CHAPTER 13 / Washing, Drying & Brushing

After conditioning, squeeze or shake out excess water, and pat your hair dry using the towel as a blotter. Do not rub your hair or you may rough up the cuticle layer surface, or break fragile hair shafts. A hairstyle for which air drying will suffice is ideal; blow dryers can damage hair if improperly used. If you must use a blow dryer, do so after you have towel-dried the hair from wet to damp. Use a dryer with power less than 1000 watts, and set it at the lowest heat level. Stop as soon as the hair is dry (or even still slightly damp). Damage is done to the hair by over-drying. A wide nozzle dryer is preferable, as it diffuses the heat more and is easier on the hair. Keep the dryer at least six inches from the hair and keep it moving, directing the air over and through the hair. The nozzle should not be directed at the scalp and hair roots.

Hair that is wet or is being blow-dried should be combed with a wide-toothed, smooth-edged comb with blunt tips. Hair swells on contact with water and becomes more fragile when wet. At this point the hair is so elastic that a brush may easily stretch and snap the hair shaft. Work out tangles by combing gently, starting from the ends and working toward the scalp.

Regular brushing is an important step in your effort to prevent hair loss and improve the quality of your hair. The pulling effect of brushing aids circulation and stimulates the scalp. It also brings oil from the roots of the hair all the way down to the ends, promoting a more lustrous look. Finally, it helps to brush out debris such as dust, dirt and flakes of dandruff.

In order to achieve deep, scalp stimulating brushing, you must work on your hair twice daily. Gently brush for three to five minutes, once in the morning and once in the evening. Brush for three minutes if your hair is short, and up to five minutes if it is longer.

Bending your head toward the floor while brushing will bring more blood flow to the head, increasing circulation to the scalp. Do not overbrush (your scalp should not feel raw and sore afterwards), or you'll risk causing 'traction alopecia,' a condition of temporary hair loss as a result of overzealous brushing.

CHAPTER 13 / Washing, Drying & Brushing

Alternate with up and down strokes. Move from the top of the head and down the sides, to the neck, sides and forehead and up towards the top of the head. Remember to start brushing at the roots of the hair; the glands of your own scalp produce the best anti-dryness grooming oil available. By completing the strokes in one movement, oil is evenly distributed. However, if you have long hair, stroke only halfway, then hold the hair with one hand and complete the stroke with the other hand holding the brush. The problem with a continuous stroke on long hair is that of placing too much stress on the hair shaft and root, which can cause breakage.

The best type of brush to use is one made of natural bristle (usually boar). Just like your hair, the bristle is made of natural keratin, and will catch dirt and debris in the same way that your hair does. The dirt is absorbed by the bristles and removed from the hair. A nylon brush will not accomplish the same cleaning process. When the natural bristle brush gets dirty, just scrub it with a dry towel, or wipe the bristles with a towel after each brushing. Natural bristles have rounded ends, which is easier on the scalp and the hair shaft than the sharp bristles found on most nylon brushes. If you do purchase a nylon brush, make sure that the bristles have rounded ends. Natural bristle brushes are commonly available in natural foods stores. Chinese community stores and certain drugstores. Wooden combs, also available in health food stores and in Chinese stores, keep out static, which can be a problem for certain types of hair.

CHAPTER 14 Nasty
Chemicles

IIT HAS BEEN ESTIMATED by some that up to 80% of all cosmetic ingredients depend in some way on petroleum for a portion of their molecular structure. To a chemist, a molecule is a molecule and it doesn't matter where it comes from. In the natural health field however, petroleum-sourced materials are considered at least debatable, if not downright dangerous. One has only to look at Vitamin E, which when derived from petroleum sources, is only half as bioavailable as natural source E and blocks E receptors in the body.

Most herbs used cosmetically are processed in propylene glycol, yet the label is not required to state this fact unless it was added in pure form to the final product. Propylene glycol is a synthetic petrochemical product linked to allergic and toxic reactions. Ingredients derived solely from petroleum include mineral oil, paraffin, petrolatum, isopropyl alcohol, microcrystalline wax and carbomers. Those ingredients that are partially petroleum-based can be identified by the inclusion of these affixes: ethyl; methyl; butyl; propyl; octyl; PVP; -ene and -eth.

These chemicals, as well as others commonly found in shampoos, conditioners, hair sprays and dyes (not to mention other personal care products) can cause a wide range of health problems, including allergic reactions, chemical sensitization, skin irritations, and cancer. Irritation is defined as an inflammatory reaction, non-allergic in nature, which occurs on the area exposed to a given substance. Inflammation appears within minutes to hours of contact. The severity of the reaction depends on the concentration of the irritant and the susceptibility of the individual. When product use is

CHAPTER 14 / Nasty Chemicles

discontinued the symptoms diminish. In the case of shampoos, inflammation occurring on the scalp can shrink the follicle openings, choking off the hair shaft, impairing the health and growth of the hair.

Allergens and sensitizers, unlike irritants, involve the immune system. While the symptoms of exposure may be similar to irritation, the reaction usually appears from 24 to 48 hours after contact, and the symptoms may increase in intensity over the next few days. The reaction may also show up any place else on the skin and may remain for days or weeks. A sensitizer may not trigger a response upon initial use, but repeated use can cause the development of an allergic reaction to even very low amounts of the chemical involved.

The leading causes of allergy, irritation and sensitization found in cosmetics and hair-care products are fragrances and preservatives. Allergy symptoms to look for include: watery eyes, reddened skin, nausea, depression, lethargy, mood swings, irritability, restlessness, anger, memory lapses and inability to concentrate. Granted, these symptoms are common, but then so are the chemicals we are discussing.

Preservatives

Preservatives are required in cosmetic products to prevent bacteria contamination and extend shelf life, but even the American Academy of Dermatology acknowledges that they are a leading cause of contact dermatitis. The worst of the preservatives release small amounts of formaldehyde, which is an allergen, irritant and sensitizer, and also a carcinogen and neurotoxin. Diazolidinyl and Imidazolidinyl Urea (also found under the trade names Germall II and Germall 115) release formaldehyde at just 10 degrees F. Other chemicals that contain, release or break down into formaldehyde include: 2-bromo-2-nitropropane-1, 3-diol; DM hydantoin; Quaternium 15.

Other preservatives, which do not contain formaldehyde but do have a greater than normal potential for causing irritation and allergic reactions include: Methylchloroisothiazolinone; Methylisothiazolinone; and the infamous Paraben family (butyl, ethyl, methyl and propyl). The Parabens, linked to skin rashes and other allergic reactions, are hard to avoid even in 'natural' shampoos and conditioners. Methyl paraben particularly should be avoided, being partially composed of benzoic acid, a substance linked to many serious ailments by Hulda Clark, in her book 'Cure For All Diseases.'

Preservatives which seem to cause the least irritation and fewest allergic reactions, yet are still effective include: Grapefruit seed extract ('Citricidal,' 'Nutribiotic'); Potassium sorbate; Sorbic acid; Tocopherol (Vit.E); Retinyl (Vit.A); Ascorbic acid (Vit.C).

Fragrance

In most fragrances 95% of the mix is made from synthetic chemicals, and a synthetic fragrance can be made up of 600 or so raw ingredients, most of which have the potential to cause an allergic or toxic response. In fact many of the chemicals used in fragrances are considered hazardous, including: Methylene chloride; Toluene; Methyl ethyl ketone; Methyl isobutyl ketone; Ethyl alcohol; and Benzyl chloride. Nevertheless, manufacturers are not obligated to disclose on the label the ingredients used in formulating their fragrances.

Roughly 84% of the ingredients used in fragrances have either never been tested, or tested only minimally for human toxicity. Yet the National Institute of Occupational Safety and Health recently reported that in a list of 2,983 chemicals used in the fragrance industry, 884 toxic substances were identified as capable of causing allergic reactions, breathing difficulties, multiple chemical sensitivities and neurotoxicity. In a 1991 report by the E.P.A., toluene was detected in every fragrance sample collected. Toluene is known to both cause asthma and trigger asthma attacks, and is also considered a neurotoxin. Toluene is found as well in furniture waxes, plastic garbage bags, inks, cat litter, hair gel and hair sprays. It would seem to be a wise choice to choose a shampoo and conditioner without overwhelming fragrance. After all, do we really need to smell like a pine forest or a pina colada?

CHAPTER 14 / Nasty Chemicals

Colors and Dyes

Synthetic colors, made from petrochemicals (coal tar), are defined on the label as FD & C or D & C, followed by a color and a number. Some, such as Blue 1 and Green 3 are known to be carcinogenic. Others, due to impurities found in commercial batches, have been shown to cause cancer both when ingested and when applied to the skin. These include D & C Red 33, F D & C Yellow 5, and F D &C Yellow 6. Some of the coal tar colors have also been found to contain heavy metals, including arsenic and lead, which are also carcinogenic.

Up to 40% of American women use permanent or semi-permanent hair dye products. This places them in at a high risk for cancer, particularly for non-Hodgkin's lymphoma, multiple myeloma, leukemia and Hodgkin's disease. There is evidence that up to 20% of all non-Hodgkin's lymphoma cases in U.S. women is directly linked to the use of hair-coloring products. Human and animal studies have implied that women who use hair dyes may also have an increased risk of breast cancer.

The black, brown/brunette and red hair dyes carry a significantly higher risk than the lighter colored dyes. Any dye using phenylenediamine-based ingredients should be considered carcinogenic. Temporary dyes and rinses that contain the chemicals Acid Orange 87, Solvent Brown 44, Acid Blue 168, and Acid Violet 73 should also be avoided as known carcinogens. Bleaches are much safer than dyes. Though they are harsh on the hair and scalp, they most likely do not pose any long-term danger. Natural hennas are a safe alternative to dyes that are actually good for the hair. There are also new dye systems out of Europe that use no coal tar colors, which can be found in health food stores.

It has been pointed out that women who start dyeing their hair at age 40 have a risk factor less than one third of those who start at age 30. Those who start at age 20 have a risk twice as great as those who started at 40. These facts obviously can be extrapolated to men who dye their hair. Due to lobbyists, hair dyes are among the most loosely regulated of all consumer products. Canadians may rest assured that they have the same level

CHAPTER 14 / Nasty Chemicles

of protection that Americans do.

Additional Cancer Risks

DEA (diethanolamine) and TEA (triethanolamine) are wetting agents, found in both mainstream and 'natural' personal care products and often bound to other compounds, such as in 'cocamide DEA' or 'TEA sodium lauryl sulphate.'

While DEA and TEA are not carcinogenic per se, if they are in the presence of nitrates, a chemical reaction occurs that forms nitrosamines, which are known carcinogens. Unfortunately the nitrates, used as a preservative or present as a byproduct, need not be disclosed on the label. Since there is no adequate label disclosure legislation, we cannot know which DEA and TEA containing products are safe, as we have no way of knowing which products also contain nitrates. One option is to choose products from Germany. Since 1987 the German Federal Health Office has discouraged their manufacturers from using DEA and TEA.

To find out about the dangerous and questionable chemicals in makeup, dental hygiene products antiperspirants and deodorants, shaving creams, skin lotions, soaps and related personal care products, we highly recommend consulting 'The Safe Shopper's Bible,' by David Steinman and Samuel Epstein. You will also find there a safety review of the most commonly available shampoos, conditioners, and other hair care products.

CHAPTER 15 The Oriental Approach

Part One: Macrobiotics

EVER SINCE THE LIKES of Charlie Chan and Bruce Lee sleuthed and kicked their ways across the movie screen, America has been increasingly fascinated by the ways of the mysterious East. From kung fu to acupuncture to the austere spiritually of Zen Buddhism, these cultural imports from afar were adopted by many a Westerner looking for something new.

One oriental tradition that continues to make inroads is its approach to health. Unlike Western medicines concern with the treatment of illness and disease, oriental medicine focuses on prevention. Health is seen as the body's natural state throughout life. As such, disease is not something we must always fight to keep at bay; it is instead a symptom of a person's lack of harmony, either within the body or with the environment. Of course one might ask: what exactly does 'harmony' mean?

The answer lies in the fact that the healing arts are not seen as a specific, separate field, but rather as part of a larger, interconnected philosophy. Finding health and harmony, then, becomes a something of a balancing act. A Japanese version of this philosophy of balance made its way to American under the moniker of macrobiotics. Its' very name, meaning the great or large (macro) way of life (biotic) indicates its philosophical scope, but it is most commonly viewed as a strict form of dietary practice derived from Zen Buddhism. The perceived strictness of Macrobiotics led to mixed reviews in its early attempts to find a toehold in America, ranging from fanatical enthusiasm to 'dangerous fringe diet' labels. It quickly proved its

CHAPTER 15 / The Oriental Approach

adaptability, however, and before long it developed a healthy following.

Authors and teachers like George Ohsawa, Michio Kushi and Herman Aihara traveled worldwide to share their message, playing a significant role in the development of the natural foods and alternative healing movements. Unlike the latest herbal remedy, however, macrobiotics is not easily encapsulated. As an all-encompassing philosophy, it is beyond the scope of one chapter but a brief examination of some of its basic ideas will allow us to see how to apply these to hair health, and hair loss prevention.

A good starting point is be the yin-yang symbol. As the image suggests, it is a symbol of balance: two relative opposites, each containing a seed of the other, in constant transformation as they move in an endless circle. We see examples of this everywhere in nature: night and day, summer and winter, male and female. By using these polarities as a kind of compass, it becomes possible to achieve some kind of 'balance.' As this system can become quite complicated, a more straightforward approach in terms of diet, is to classify foods in terms of pH-acidity or alkalinity –and the effects they have on the body.

Central to this dietary practice is what is known as the 'standard macrobiotic diet.' In terms of yin and yang, these foods sit pretty close to the middle – not too acidic, not too alkaline –so they are considered safe foods for daily consumption. They are preferably locally grown, or at least grown in climate conditions similar to those in your area. For those of us in temperate zones this means the majority of our diet should consist of whole grains (e.g. wheat, rice, oats), beans and certain vegetables, supplemented with fish, sea vegetables, nuts and seeds. As we move towards the more extreme foods, the balancing act becomes more complicated, so that for optimal health it is recommended that these foods be avoided.

A quick glance at the more yin and yang foods might leave you saying "...that's all fine, but there is nothing good left to eat!" Most of our favorite foods fall into either extreme. The key point to remember, however, is balance, and thinking in these terms might still prove useful for health, especially when there are some things that you don't want to give up. For exam-

CHAPTER 15 / The Oriental Approach

ple, having a bit of cheese (yang) with that glass of wine (yin) balances things out quite nicely.

To illustrate how these principles apply to hair loss some macrobiotic teachers will compare hair to a growing plant. Hair loss is related to the condition of the scalp, which is compared to the soil in which the plant grows. If the soil is too moist and watery (yin), the plant doesn't grown deep roots; it is uprooted easily. Conversely, if the soil is too dry and sandy (yang), the plant is again easily removed.

There are different ways of finding out whether we have too much yin or too much yang (it is possible to have both). Most obviously we can observe our diet. Accomplished macrobiotic practitioners uses a more sophisticated technique known as oriental diagnosis, an ancient method used in many eastern healing practices. This involves observing the many characteristics that make us unique individuals, from posture and physique to skin tone, facial features, pulse and quality of voice. Each of these is said to reflect some kinds of internal state, such as blood quality or the health of an organ. By putting all of this together, a person condition becomes apparent to the trained practitioner.

Oriental medicine relates the condition of the hair to the condition of the intestines. Where you lose your hair, however, is indicative of how you are imbalanced: hair loss towards the top and front of the head indicates too much yin, especially sweets, fruits and alcohol. Hair loss at the crown indicates excessive yang, notably salt and animal protein. An interesting correspondence between this view and modern medicine is that too much cholesterol can raise levels of DHT, the "bad" testosterone, leading to male pattern baldness at the top of the head. High cholesterol stems from over-consumption of foods like meat and eggs –in other words, too much yang.

The natural approach of macrobiotics also offers some techniques to help prevent hair loss and perhaps even stimulate new growth. One such treatment is the pine needle scalp massage. This method requires a bundle of fresh pine needles, approximately one inch in diameter, bound up in a pen shape. The scalp is stimulated by poking it gently, increasing blood circu-

CHAPTER 15 / The Oriental Approach

lation. Short periods of use each day gradually strengthen the skin and help bring nutrients to hair follicles. It is also possible that some pine oil is imparted to the scalp, which may have its own usefulness: France's Pasteur Institute has shown this invigorating oil to have strong antiseptic activity. Following the massage it is recommended that you vigorously rub a mixture of fresh, raw ginger juice and sesame oil (in a 1:1 ratio), a nourishing and stimulating combination similar to those recommended elsewhere in this book.

The appeal of macrobiotics for supporting hair health may lie in its sheer practicality. Its dietary focus encourages self-reliance in healing and makes it markedly less expensive than many other prevention techniques. Using food to heal is nothing new, nor is it exclusively Eastern –the father of Western medicine, Hippocrates, once said, "Let food be thy medicine." In modern times, this seemingly radical message is as accessible and as flexible as it was two thousand years ago. If the macrobiotic approach is correct, it is indeed possible to prevent hair loss and even re-grow hair through diet alone. What could be simpler?

Foods most YIN	*Foods most YANG*
chemicals	**seeds**
alcohol	**root vegetables**
coffee	**sea vegetables**
sugar	**beans**
honey	**whole grains**
spices	**fish**
butter & oils	**poultry**
tropical fruits	**cheese**
nightshade plants	**red meat**
(tomato, potato, eggplant)	**eggs**
local fruits and nuts	**salt**
leafy greens	

CHAPTER 15 / The Oriental Approach

Part Two: The Chinese Approach

Explaining the entire Chinese approach to medicine to the unacquainted Western mind requires the length of books, not chapters. But with space constraints in mind, we will jump right into the middle and hope those who might want more information, will be sufficiently stimulated to acquire it. In the bibliography you will find some books listed that are a good place to find more information on the subject.

In Oriental tradition the human is a microcosm of nature, an inseparable manifestation of nature as people. We represent the offspring of heaven and Earth: a fusion of cosmic and terrestrial forces. Nature is a single unified system, as symbolized by the Tao: the opposing and complementary aspects of Yin and Yang. Life flows with harmony when the elements of Nature are in balance, and when the balance is upset there is 'dis'-ease. This is the philosophical base from which the very practical methods of Chinese medicine stem.

The vocabulary of Chinese medicine includes metaphors from Nature such as; Wood, Fire, Earth, Metal, Water, Heat, Wind and Cold. While these words have specific meaning in the Chinese medical system only, the West shares the terminology that refers to the organs. For example, both systems will use words like deficient to describe a condition of the kidney. In Chinese medicine, however, a deficient kidney cannot be strictly interpreted as a weak kidney.

This is because Chinese medicine defines the organs functionally, not structurally. In the west, when we refer to the kidney we simply mean that particular organ and nothing else. The Chinese system, however, is based on organ networks. The Kidney refers not only to the organ itself, but the meridians or pathways that run through the organs, along which acupuncture points are located. This is how, for example, a Chinese doctor can locate a problem with a patient's liver by looking at the condition of the eyes. Because the eyes are part of the liver organ network.

Using this network system a single symptom is observed in relationship to

CHAPTER 15 / The Oriental Approach

the entire body environment, and problems are not isolated from the context in which they occur. It is interesting to note that while these pathway systems were charted some 5000 years ago, Western science has only recently been able to create electronics sensitive enough to detect and verify the electrical vortex present at each acupuncture point.

To the Oriental medical system, hair is considered to be an extension of the 'Blood' (capitalizing the name of the organ is to imply the organ's network. In the case of Blood, this includes the entire process of generating, distributing, and storing nutrients). The condition of the hair is one indicator of the quality of the Blood. By improving the quality of Blood and strengthening the Spleen-Pancreas and Kidneys we can begin to address the problems of hair loss and prematurely gray hair. Healthy hair also depends on sufficient blood being stored in the Liver. When Liver-Blood is deficient it is unable to rise and nourish the head.

Traditionally, the Chinese have used hijiki seaweed (a member of the kelp family), nettles (commonly used in the European tradition as well) and wheat grass to keep hair from falling out and to prevent gray hair. These foods are rich in Blood-building chlorophyll (the nettles and wheat grass), and all will detoxify the blood.

You may have heard of the Chinese herb Ho Shou Wu, also known as Fo Ti in North America (Polygonum Muliflorum). Fo Ti is a traditional tonic for restoring gray hair, and is considered a general rejuvenator and longevity agent. Fo Ti has been marketed to Westerners in formulas promising to re-grow lost hair. At least one modern Chinese text (Healing With Whole Foods by Paul Pitchford) however, suggests that Fo Ti is too warming and tonifying to the Liver for most Westerners, causing depression and anger in many cases.

That book recommends it only for those who were raised on low-fat, low-meat diets, who do not show signs of an "excessive liver" (i.e. eye problems, excessive irritability and anger, or deep vertical lines between the eyebrows).

CHAPTER 15 / The Oriental Approach

The Chinese system supports the thesis of this book: that the standard Western diet is at least partly to blame for the current epidemic of hair loss, and general poor health of the hair. It confirms that the high-fat, high-protein diet common in America acidifies the blood and damages the Kidneys. Meat and dairy products are considered "sweet" (i.e. Yin) in Chinese medicine, and when added to the high consumption of desserts and sugar-laden food and drink common in the West, reveal a typical diet unbalanced in favor of the Yin foods.

The 'Yellow Emperors Classic of Internal Medicine,' revered by Chinese healers for more than 3000 years, advises that 'too much sweet-flavored foods make the head hair fall out.' Though, lest we forget the principles of balance found in both Japanese and Chinese medicine, the Inner Classic also points out that 'too much salt damages the blood' and therefore the hair.

The spleen-pancreas, whose function is to produce blood and assimilate nutrients, is most readily affected by worry and anxiety. In China this is called 'excessive thinking.' Because worry weakens the blood, which carries the nutrients necessary for cell regeneration, it accelerates aging in general. Eating meals with simple combinations of whole foods helps produce deeper, less busy thinking. Meditation and relaxed awareness leads to less worry and stress.

Chinese doctors use acupuncture and moxibustion (using heat rather than needles to stimulate the points) in the treatment of hair loss, but the process is not as simple as describing a few points that you can use at home. It is best for one choosing this approach to find an experienced practitioner to work with, as a degree of personalization is involved. Acupuncture treatment is not fixed but is determined by the characteristic of each individual patient.

The strategy for treatment is based on the location of the patient's weaknesses, time of year, time of day, patient's work environment and daily habits. It is then modified based on things like degree of overall progress, shifting symptoms, the color and texture of the tongue, the nature of pulse, and the tone and timbre of the voice.

CHAPTER 15 / The Oriental Approach

Herbal formulas are often tailored to the individual and modified to follow his changing patterns. But Chinese medicine does have general formulas to meet common illness patterns that are uncomplicated by individual idiosyncrasies. One such formula is the 'Seven Treasures Special Pill for Beautiful Whiskers' from the Analytic collection of Medical Formulas.

This remedy is designed to 'enrich Kidney Yin and nourish the Liver-Blood.' The treatable symptoms are general enough to include premature graying of the hair or hair loss, loose teeth, nocturnal and spontaneous emissions, soreness and weakness of the lower back, declining libido, dry eyes, or unsatisfying sleep.

Kidney Essence maintains tissue and blood, elasticity of skin and muscle, and agility of the mind and clarity of the senses. The above symptoms indicate that depleted Kidney reserves have precipitated a deficiency of the blood of the liver and heart.

The commercial pre-made version of the 'Seven Treasures' formula can be found in Chinese herbal stores, but because this formula does contain 'Ho Shou Wu,' remember the warning issued earlier.

Conclusion

REMEMBER, preventing, halting or reversing hair loss is not an overnight affair. It may take months before improvements are noted, and could take a year before any new growth is apparent. In any case there are no guarantees. The key to success is daily hair care, a must for anyone with problem scalp or hair.

A condition that took a lifetime to develop cannot be reversed in a matter of days or weeks. The techniques you choose to apply must be used consistently and rigorously. Haphazard, occasional therapy will have little or no effect.

In attempting to prevent or reverse hair loss it is wise to think in terms of synergy---the whole is greater than the sun of its parts. The more multi-layered your approach the greater your chances of success.

Eliminating the causative factors under your control (e.g. smoking, excess salt consumption, excess cholesterol, high stress levels), combined with dietary changes, nutritional supplementation, scalp stimulation, externally applied formulas, and proper hair care and hygiene, can accomplish far more than any isolated approach or technique.

You are the experiment, and you are biochemically unique. Therefore a certain amount of trial and error is inevitable. To conclude we shall detail a basic routine designed to minimize hair loss, including both internal and external remedies. Of course, some personalization is necessary. Find the combination that works best for you and stick with it.

Conclusion

External

Follicle cleaning is critical to preventing fallage. While Polysorbate 80 has the best researched track record, it is somewhat awkward to apply. Jojoba Oil performs the same function of cleansing the follicles and is much easier to use, as it can be left on all night, doesn't stain, and washes out easily. It also regulates sebum production, preventing the scalp from becoming too dry or too oily, and revitalizes the hair shaft. Rosemary or peppermint oil may be added to the jojoba oil to stimulate circulation.

For a deeper cleaning action try alternating jojoba oil with apple cider vinegar. Apple cider vinegar should rubbed into the scalp at full strength, and left on for fifteen minutes before shampooing. Cider vinegar normalizes the acid mantle on the scalp and kills off any bad bacteria that may be breeding in the buildup of dead skin cells.

Circulation: Bending over from the waist and gently brushing the entire scalp will enhance circulation and clean dead skin and debris which clogs the follicles from the scalp. If you have dead cell buildup on the scalp, flaking, and/or itchy scalp it is important to shampoo regularly to aid in keeping the follicles unplugged.

Internal

Vegetal Silica: 500 mg, three per day (providing 30mg elemental silica).
Saw Palmetto Berry Extract: 160 mg Standardized Extract...twice a day if you have prostate problems, once per day if you do not.
Vitamin A: (5000 iu) with Beta Carotene (25,000 iu). Specify natural source.
Vitamin C: At least 500 mg per day. Specify 'Buffered.'
Vitamin E: At least 400 iu per day. Specify 'Natural Source.'
A multi-mineral complex that includes Calcium, Magnesium, Zinc and trace minerals.

Nothing so effectively prevents hair loss due to breakage as Vegetal Silica. Take Saw Palmetto Berry Extract for its proven ability to prevent the for-

Conclusion

mation of DHT. The three vitamins (A, C, E) are the best researched and proven antioxidants. By scavenging the free radicals that cause cellular degeneration they naturally ward off cancer and heart disease, and also help prevent premature aging and the attendant hair loss. Vitamin C also supports the function of the adrenal glands, helping to combat the excess androgens produced by these glands when under stress. Calcium and Magnesium aid in stress prevention. Zinc helps to prevent the conversion of testosterone to DHT. All other major macro minerals should be presented along with trace minerals.

Essential Fatty Acids

Essential Fatty Acids are best taken in the form of Flax seed and Fish body oils. Try to use good quality products like BARLEAN's Organic, currently available all over the US. Alternate or take them together: For example, take a tablespoon of Flax oil with your breakfast oatmeal, and a few Fish oil caps with dinner. Take supplements or eat fish at least three times per week. Omega 3 EFAs are found predominantly in the deep-water fish including salmon, herring, mackerel, trout, or sardines.

EFAs support immune functions, prevent premature aging, and regulate sebum functions, keeping the skin and hair healthy and vibrant. Because of the link between fats, EFAs, and the formation of DHT, surrounding prostate problems and Male Pattern Baldness, this is perhaps the most important area in which to exercise dietary controls. In order to raise and maintain adequate EFA levels one must also restrict the intake of 'bad' fats.

Bibliography

Adams, Ruth with Murry, Frank
  Body, Mind, and B-Vitamins (Fourth Edition):
  Los Angeles, Pinnacle Book 1972

Aihara, Cornilia and Herman, Natural Healing from Head to Toe:
  New York: Avery Publishing Group Inc., 1994

Airola, Paavo, Stop Hair Loss (Twelfth Edition):
  Phoenix, Health Plus Publishers, 1965

Balch, James F.M.D., with Balch, Phyllis A.,
  CNC, Prescription for Nutritional Healing:
  New York, Avery Publication Group, 1990

Barolet, Randall, with Bensky, Dan,
  Chinese Herbal Medicine Formulas:
  Seattle, Eastland Press, 1990

Beinfield, Harriet and Korngold, Efrem, Between Heaven and Earth:
  A Guide to Chinese Medicine: New York, Ballantine, 1991

Berry, Neville, The World's Greatest Collection of Hair Loss Remedies:
  Glan Publication, 1990

Bragg, Paul C., with Bragg, Patricia,
  Apple Cider Vinegar Health System:
  Santa Barbara, Health Science, 1990

Bibliography

Calbom, Cherie, Juicing for Life:
New York, Avery Publishing Group, 1992

Chaitow, Leon, Prostate Troubles:
London, Thorson's Publishing Group, 1988

Chapman, J.B., M.D. and Perry, Edward L., M.D.,
The Biochemical Handbook: St. Louis, Formur Publishing 1976

Dunne, Lavon J., Nutrition Almanac (Third Edition):
New York, McGraw Hill, 1990

Hampton, Aubrey, Natural Ingredients Dictionary: Florida, Organica Press, 1994

Hanssen, Maurice, The Healing Power of Pollen (Fourth Edition):
London, Thorson Pub., 1979

Heinerman, John, Aloe Vera, Jojoba, and Yucca:
Connecticut, Keats Publishing 1982

Kaufman, Klaus, Silica, The Forgotten Nutrient:
Burnaby, B.C., Alive books, 1990

Khalsa, Siri, Nutrition News Volume Eight, Number Twelve:
Pomona, Ca., 1985

Kloss, Jethro, Back to Eden: New York, Benedict Lust Pub., 1971

Kushi, Michio, The Macrobiotic Way of Natural Healing: Boston, East West Publications, 1978

Kushi, Michio, The Book of Macrobiotics: Tokyo and New York, Japan Publications Inc., 1986

Lee, William H., The Book of Raw Fruits and Vegetable Juices and

Bibliography

Drinks: Conneticut, Keats Publishing, 1982

Linde, Shirley, The Whole Health Catalogue (Third Edition): Ottawa, McClelland and Stewart, 1977

Lu, Henry C., Chinese Foods for Longevity: New York, Sterling Publishing, 1990

Lucas, Richard, Nature's Medicines (Fourth Edition): New York, Award Books, 1966

Lust, John B., The Herb Book (Thirteenth Edition): New York, Bantam Books, 1980

Lust, Benedict, Drink Your Troubles Away: New York, Benedict Lust Publications, 1967

Mindell, Earl, Vitamin Bible: New York, Warner Books, 1985

Morgan, Dr. Brian L., with Morgan, Roberta, Hormones: Los Angeles, The Body Press, 1989

Pearson, Durk, with Shaw, Sandy, Life Extension: New York, Warner Books, 1982

Pitchford, Paul, Healing With Whole Foods: Berkeley, CA, North Atlantic Books, 1993

Robbins, John, Diet for a New America: Walpole, New Hampshire, Stillpoint Pub., 1987

Segal, Darryl R., Hair For Life (Third Edition): Richmond, B.C., Copyright By the Author, 1984

Stein, Irene, Royal Jelly: London, Thorson's Pub., 1989

Bibliography

Steinman, David and Epstein, Samuel, M.D., The Safe Shoppers Bible: New York, MacMillan, 1995

Tenney, Louise, Today's Herbal Health (Second Edition): Utah, Woodland Books, 1983

Tierra, Michael, The Way of Herbs: Santa Cruz, Unity Press, 1980

Trattler, Dr. Ross, Better Health Through Natural Healing: New York, McGraw-Hill, 1985

Treben, Maria, Health From God's Garden: Vermont, Healing Arts Press, 1985

Vogel, A, M.D., Swiss Nature Doctor (Forty Fourth Edition): Switzerland, 1952

Wade, Carlson, Magic Minerals: New York Parker Publishing, 1967

Wade, Carlson, Natural Hormones: The Secret of Youthful Health: New York, Parker Publishing, 1972

Weller, Stella, Super Healthy Hair, Skin and Nails: London, Harper Collins, 1991

For these and other titles on health visit:
www.applepublishing.com